Immunizations

Editor

MARGOT SAVOY

PRIMARY CARE: CLINICS IN OFFICE PRACTICE

www.primarycare.theclinics.com

Consulting Editor
JOEL J. HEIDELBAUGH

September 2020 • Volume 47 • Number 3

ELSEVIER

1600 John F. Kennedy Boulevard • Suite 1800 • Philadelphia, Pennsylvania, 19103-2899

http://www.theclinics.com

PRIMARY CARE: CLINICS IN OFFICE PRACTICE Volume 47, Number 3
September 2020 ISSN 0095-4543, ISBN-13: 978-0-323-75579-5

Editor: Katerina Heidhausen
Developmental Editor: Laura Fisher

Primary Care: Clinics in Office Practice (ISSN: 0095-4543) is published quarterly by Elsevier Inc., 360 Park Avenue South, New York, NY 10010-1710. Months of issue are March, June, September, and December. Periodicals postage paid at New York, NY and additional mailing offices. Subscription prices are $253.00 per year (US individuals), $538.00 (US institutions), $100.00 (US students), $303.00 (Canadian individuals), $609.00 (Canadian institutions), $100.00 (Canadian students), $357.00 (international individuals), $609.00 (international institutions), and $175.00 (international students). Foreign air speed delivery is included in all *Clinics* subscription prices. All prices are subject to change without notice. POSTMASTER: Send address changes to *Primary Care: Clinics in Office Practice*, Elsevier Periodicals Customer Service, 11830 Westline Industrial Drive, St. Louis, MO 63146. Customer Service Health Sciences Division, Subscription Customer Service, 3251 Riverport Lane, Maryland Heights, MO 63043. **Customer Service: 1-800-654-2452 (U.S. and Canada); 314-447-8871 (outside U.S. and Canada). Fax: 314-447-8029. E-mail: journalscustomerservice-usa@elsevier.com (for print support); journalsonlinesupport-usa@elsevier.com (for online support).**

Reprints. For copies of 100 or more, of articles in this publication, please contact the Commercial Reprints Department, Elsevier Inc., 360 Park Avenue South, New York, NY 10010-1710. Tel. 212-633-3874; Fax: 212-633-3820; E-mail: reprints@elsevier.com.

Primary Care: Clinics in Office Practice is covered in *MEDLINE/PubMed (Index Medicus) and EMBASE/Excerpta Medica, Current Contents/Clinical Medicine, and ISI/BIOMED.*

Contributors

CONSULTING EDITOR

JOEL J. HEIDELBAUGH, MD, FAAFP, FACG
Clinical Professor, Departments of Family Medicine and Urology, Director of Medical Student Education and Clerkship Director, Department of Family Medicine, University of Michigan Medical School, Ann Arbor, Michigan; Ypsilanti Health Center, Ypsilanti, Michigan

EDITOR

MARGOT SAVOY, MD, MPH, FAAFP, FABC, CPE, CMQ, FAAPL
Department Chair and Associate Professor, Family and Community Medicine, Chief Quality Officer, Temple Faculty Practice, Lewis Katz School of Medicine, Temple University, Philadelphia, Pennsylvania

AUTHORS

SARAH COLES, MD
Assistant Professor, Department of Family, Community and Preventive Medicine, Family Medicine Residency, University of Arizona College of Medicine - Phoenix, Phoenix, Arizona

JOHN W. EPLING, MD, MSEd
Professor, Department of Family and Community Medicine, Virginia Tech Carilion School of Medicine, Roanoke, Virginia

JENNIFER L. HAMILTON, MD, PhD
Associate Professor, Department of Family, Community, and Preventive Medicine, Drexel University College of Medicine, Philadelphia, Pennsylvania

ERIN KAVANAUGH, MD, FAAFP
Vice Chair, Clinical Assistant Professor, Department of Family and Community Medicine, Program Director, Family Medicine Residency, Co-Program Director, Emergency Medicine/Family Medicine Residency, Sidney Kimmel Medical College, Christiana Care Health System, Wilmington, Delaware

MINA S. KHAN, MD, FAAFP
Family Medicine, Primary Care Services-Blount, LLC, Oneonta, Alabama

JAMIE LOEHR, MD, FAAFP
Owner, Cayuga Family Medicine, Ithaca, New York

MELISSA L. MARTINEZ, MD
Professor, Department of Internal Medicine, University of New Mexico, Health Sciences Center, Albuquerque, New Mexico

RANIT MISHORI, MD, MHS, FAAFP
Professor of Family Medicine, Director Global Heath Initiatives, Department of Family Medicine, Georgetown University School of Medicine, Washington, DC

LAURA MORRIS, MD, MSPH, FAAFP
Associate Professor, Department of Family and Community Medicine, University of Missouri School of Medicine, Columbia, Missouri

DAVID O'GUREK, MD, FAAFP
Associate Professor, Department of Family and Community Medicine, Lewis Katz School of Medicine, Temple University, Philadelphia, Pennsylvania

ORITSETSEMAYE OTUBU, MD, MPH, FAAFP
Physician, MedStar Urgent Care, Washington, DC

AMRA A. RESIC, MD, FAAFP
Family Medicine Physician, Department of Family Medicine, BayCare Medical Group, Palm Harbor, Florida

MARGOT SAVOY, MD, MPH, FAAFP, FABC, CPE, CMQ, FAAPL
Department Chair and Associate Professor, Family and Community Medicine, Chief Quality Officer, Temple Faculty Practice, Lewis Katz School of Medicine, Temple University, Philadelphia, Pennsylvania

ALEXANDRA SCHIEBER, DO
Assistant Professor, Department of Family and Community Medicine, Lewis Katz School of Medicine, Temple University, Philadelphia, Pennsylvania

MARY M. STEPHENS, MD, MPH, FAAFP
Associate Professor, Department of Family and Community Medicine, Jefferson University Hospitals, Philadelphia, Pennsylvania

SARAH SWOFFORD, MD, MSPH
Associate Professor, Department of Family and Community Medicine, University of Missouri School of Medicine, Columbia, Missouri

Contents

Foreword: The World Has Changed **xi**

Joel J. Heidelbaugh

Preface: The Immunization Conundrum **xiii**

Margot Savoy

Establishing and Maintaining a Vaccine-Positive Practice Culture **395**

Amra A. Resic

A vaccine-positive practice culture encourages immunization against vaccine-preventable diseases by supporting policies and practices that reduce barriers and improve efficacy for vaccine delivery. Key components of a vaccine-positive practice include a well-trained, knowledgeable, collaborative health care practice team; access to immunizations in the practice; and a vaccine practice champion. Leveraging these encourages a provaccine environment and fosters productive dialogue, even among vaccine-hesitant patients/parents.

Creating a Sustainable Vaccine Delivery Practice **407**

Jamie Loehr

Providing vaccines places a significant logistical and financial burden on an office but is important in providing care to patients. Start the process by finding a vaccine champion, choosing a primary and backup vaccine coordinator, and creating a team in the office to promote and administer vaccines. Follow best practices when storing and monitoring vaccines. Create office policies for ordering vaccines in a fiscally sound manner, accepting deliveries, and managing inventory. Have backup processes in place to avoid preventable errors when administering vaccines. In addition, bill vaccine administration codes appropriately to collect the full reimbursement that is due.

Communicating About Immunizations **419**

Jamie Loehr

A significant minority of patients and parents are vaccine hesitant, defined as having the desire to delay or defer immunizations despite easy access to vaccines. Vaccine hesitancy exists along a spectrum, from patients who are concerned but willing to accept the recommended vaccine schedule to those who wish to use a delayed schedule to those who refuse vaccines altogether. A strong recommendation in favor of a vaccine is the most important reason a patient or parent accepts the immunization. Structural changes, such as removing personal and religious exemptions for vaccines required for attending school, are effective tools in increasing vaccination rates.

Vaccine Safety 431

Laura Morris and Sarah Swofford

The details of vaccine development, licensing, and monitoring have never been more important and relevant to the health care conversation in the United States. The potential exists for a preventive medicine such as a vaccine to cause harm, and physicians and patients need to understand the real balance of risks and benefits of immunization. Vaccines given in the United States undergo rigorous testing before licensure as well as extensive postlicensure safety monitoring.

Vaccinating in Pregnancy: Opportunities and Challenges 443

Alexandra Schieber and David O'Gurek

The continuum of preconception, antenatal period, fourth trimester, and interconception period are a critical time for comprehensive care to advance maternal-child health and deliver family-centered care. Immunizations are a key component of this care delivery; however, there are intricacies around indications of vaccinations during this key period. Both active immunity to the individual receiving the vaccine as well as passive immunity passed to the fetus during pregnancy highlight the benefits of this care. Understanding the indications and benefits of vaccine administration during this continuum is critical for providers caring for individuals of reproductive age.

Improving Immunization Coverage in Special Populations 453

Mary M. Stephens and Erin Kavanaugh

This highlights the key recommendations for immunization in the setting of chronic disease, children and adults with special needs, and health care providers. Immunization is an effective strategy to reduce the burden of suffering and cost of care from chronic disease. Standard child and adolescent and adult immunization schedules identify categories of high-risk conditions and chronic diseases. Clinicians need to develop systems to evaluate patients' risk factors and tailor immunization recommendations to their individual needs. Patients with intellectual disabilities, neurologic and neurodevelopmental disorders, and autism are at higher risk for vaccine-preventable illness and face significant health disparities.

Recognizing Vaccine-Preventable Diseases and Managing Outbreaks 467

Jennifer L. Hamilton

Outbreaks of vaccine-preventable diseases are becoming more common in the United States. Outbreaks of some diseases, such as measles, can be attributed to decreasing vaccination rates. Clinicians need to be aware of the vulnerabilities in their communities. Detection of an outbreak requires familiarity with signs, symptoms, and laboratory findings for these now unusual diseases. Clinicians also need to work with public health officials to identify, treat, and limit the spread of these infections. This article describes the populations most at risk from illnesses associated with sporadic outbreaks, with information on diagnosis, treatment, and ways to limit the spread of infection.

Addressing Immunization Health Disparities 483

Melissa L. Martinez and Sarah Coles

Vaccines can prevent illness but are effective only if they reach a majority of the population at risk. Disparities based on many factors, such as race and ethnicity, economic status, and rural versus urban locations of residents, are ongoing issues in the United States. Reasons for disparities include cost, access, coverage, attitudes/beliefs, and systems issues. At the government level, programs like Vaccines for Children, Medicaid reform, Medicare, and state efforts funded in part by 317 grants have helped reduce but not eliminate disparities. At a practice level, vaccine disparities can be addressed by community outreach and systems to offer and deliver vaccines.

Immunizing in a Global Society: Vaccines for Travelers 497

Oritsetsemaye Otubu and Ranit Mishori

The risk of travel-related illnesses that require vaccines varies depending on destination and traveler characteristics. Travelers who are not immune and going to countries and regions with endemic diseases are at risk of contracting vaccine-preventable diseases; they can serve as conduits of the disease on return to their home country. Individual travelers can work with a health care professional to assess travel risk based on diseases endemic to the region, time of year of travel, and presence of acute outbreaks. Travelers should discuss personal medical history, immunization status, purpose of trip, and other individual risk factors to help determine which vaccines they need.

What's New in Vaccine Science 517

Margot Savoy

Today vaccines can provide immunity against and treatment of a growing number of diseases including noninfectious conditions. Vaccine science continues to evolve newer and safer ways to deliver prevention and treatment of infectious and noninfectious diseases. This includes new adjuvants to enhance immunogenicity; delivery systems to reduce pain and improve acceptability; a wider range of uses including preventing emerging infectious diseases, such as Zika virus and Ebola, treatment of chronic diseases, such as cancer, and autoimmune disorders; and repurposing of existing vaccines, such as bacillus Calmette-Guérin for novel therapies.

Impact of Human Papillomavirus Vaccination in Reducing Cancer 529

Mina S. Khan and Margot Savoy

Human papillomavirus (HPV) is a significant cause of global morbidity and mortality. A nonavalent HPV vaccine is widely available and recommended for routine use at 11 to 12 years old. Older teens and adults though age 45 years also could be offered vaccination. Widespread use of the HPV vaccine appears to impact the rate of infections and cancers. Some parents/teens may hesitate to be vaccinated. The strongest predictor to receiving the vaccine remains a trusted health care professional making a strong

recommendation to receive the vaccine. New HPV vaccines are in the pipeline, including therapeutic vaccines to treat HPV-related cancers.

Vaccine Policy in the United States **539**

John W. Epling

In an era when the success of the US vaccination policies to date is threatened by vaccine hesitancy, it is important for clinicians to have a working understanding of how vaccines are developed and recommended for use in the United States and how federal and state governments are coordinated to ensure a safe and effective vaccine supply. This article discusses the federal agencies involved in vaccine development and recommendation, other organizations involved in vaccine policy, and the role of vaccine-related public health law in promoting universal vaccination.

PRIMARY CARE: CLINICS IN OFFICE PRACTICE

FORTHCOMING ISSUES

December 2020
Nephrology
Parvathi Perumareddi, *Editor*

March 2021
Immigrant Health
Fern R. Hauck and Carina Brown, *Editors*

June 2021
LGBTQ+ Health
Jessica Lapinski and Kristine Diaz, *Editors*

RECENT ISSUES

June 2020
Adolescent Medicine
Benjamin Silverberg, *Editor*

March 2020
Sports Medicine
Peter J. Carek, *Editor*

December 2019
Population Health
Devdutta G. Sangvai and Anthony J. Viera, *Editors*

Foreword
The World Has Changed

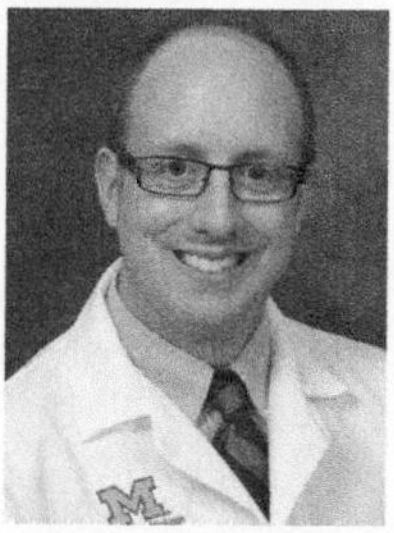

Joel J. Heidelbaugh, MD, FAAFP, FACG
Consulting Editor

I am very privileged to have been the consulting editor of *Primary Care: Clinics in Office Practice* since 2007 and am honored to continue serving our readers. Like my colleague consulting editors across the many other *Clinics* series, we strive to provide key topics for each issue coupled with relevant subtopics authored by leading experts. This issue on immunizations is no different. Yet since our plan to create this important issue, the world has changed. Forever.

Since the preproduction of this issue began, the world has been struck by the COVID-19 pandemic. It is now mid-May 2020, some 2 months after the explosion of this health care crisis in the United States, and we are still on lockdown. While we pray that the pandemic dies out and we reopen America for business very soon, it appears that we have a race to end this nightmare and prevent a second wave of illness and death: will herd immunity offer prevention first or will we have a viable vaccine? Moreover, if we have a vaccine for COVID-19, will it be widely available to all people? Will people want it or reject it? Will it be as polarizing as the yearly influenza vaccine? The answers to these questions are yet to be determined, but are extremely important on all levels and for all populations.

Prior to COVID-19, health care providers have seen increasing trends in immunization refusal. We struggle to provide education to parents, children, adolescents, and families to change their minds. This issue of *Primary Care: Clinics in Office Practice* highlights articles dedicated to establishing a positive immunization practice culture while creating a sustainable vaccine delivery practice. The issue outlines safety in immunizations, scientific evidence behind vaccines, and current policies across various populations of individuals and conditions while addressing disparities.

I would like to congratulate and thank Dr Margot Savoy and her expert authors for creating an important body of work on immunization practices. The articles herein not only provide salient guidelines for health care practitioners but also address challenges, barriers, and strategies for successful immunization practices. Prior to reading

Prim Care Clin Office Pract 47 (2020) xi–xii
https://doi.org/10.1016/j.pop.2020.06.002

this issue, I believe we all recognized the importance of immunization to prevent horrible diseases and disastrous outcomes. After reading these articles, it is apparent that we must band together as a global community to understand vaccine safety, provide available immunizations and appropriate education, and deftly manage widespread outbreaks.

Joel J. Heidelbaugh, MD, FAAFP, FACG
Departments of Family Medicine and Urology
University of Michigan Medical School
Ann Arbor, MI, USA

Ypsilanti Health Center
200 Arnet, Suite 200
Ypsilanti, MI 48198, USA

E-mail address:
jheidel@umich.edu

Preface
The Immunization Conundrum

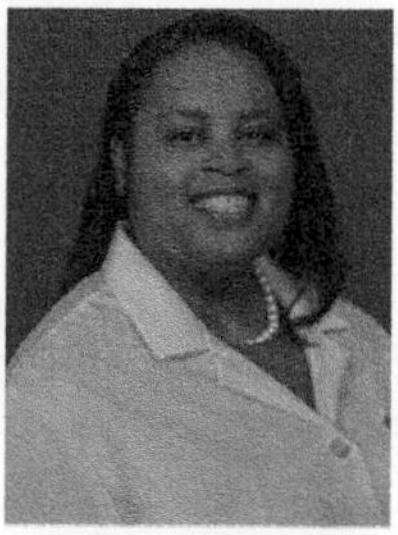

Margot Savoy, MD, MPH, FAAFP, FABC, CPE, CMQ, FAAPL
Editor

It is an intriguing time to be a vaccine science expert. At our fingertips is a wealth of safe, effective vaccines to prevent disease. We have expanding knowledge of how to identify those in greatest need and tailor the schedules to maximize their benefit in special populations. We leverage growing understanding of maternal immunity to boost immunity in our vulnerable infants, protecting them from deadly infectious diseases. We have access to rapidly advancing technology poised to transform immunization from a mechanism primarily to prevent infectious contagious disease to one that could treat and prevent chronic diseases. Finding an immunization solution to cancer or diabetes will be as game-changing to medical science as eradicating smallpox was in 1980.

Through all this success and triumph, we continue to find ourselves mired in familiar controversies and struggling to protect communities in our society. On-going hesitancy and resistance to immunization fueled by Internet-connected influencers promoting questionable claims are sparking growing outbreaks of previously eliminated communicable diseases. Hurried clinicians lacking sustainable reimbursement models struggle to find time to adequately tackle the rising number of questions in a routine office visit and miss opportunities to leverage their critical communication skills, engaging in meaningful dialogue and shared decision making about vaccine choices. Health disparities seen in immunization offers and receipt of vaccine may be related not only to differential access to health care but also to other social determinants of health and cultural factors, such as an on-going distrust of the medical establishment in communities harmed in the not-so-distant past. On-going global and national policies continue to be debated over vaccine exemptions, immunization coverage required to enter a country, and who/how vaccines should be financed.

And yet there remains hope. Clinicians no longer need to carry the burden of vaccine education and promotion alone. Team-based care strategies not only support the development of a vaccine-positive culture through education and team empowerment,

Prim Care Clin Office Pract 47 (2020) xiii–xiv
https://doi.org/10.1016/j.pop.2020.06.001
0095-4543/20/© 2020 Published by Elsevier Inc.

but with leadership development and support a vaccine champion can transform your practice. The human papilloma virus vaccine, hindered with unfounded fears around side effects, sexual promiscuity, and unconscious bias around cervical cancer risk, has already begun to markedly reduce the risk of developing cervical cancer in the countries where it was implemented widely. A cancer vaccine that is delivering on the promise of preventing cancer! The future of immunization is bright.

It was truly a pleasure to work with the outstanding vaccine science experts who contributed to this issue of *Primary Care: Clinics in Office Practice*. I hope you enjoy reading it as much as we enjoyed writing it!

Margot Savoy, MD, MPH, FAAFP, FABC, CPE, CMQ, FAAPL
Lewis Katz School of Medicine
Temple University
1316 West Ontario Street, Room 310
Philadelphia, PA 19140, USA

E-mail address:
Margot.Savoy@tuhs.temple.edu

Establishing and Maintaining a Vaccine-Positive Practice Culture

Amra A. Resic, MD*

KEYWORDS

- Vaccine hesitancy • Immunization advocacy • Cultural competency
- Vaccine champion • Decision making • Vaccine-positive practice culture

KEY POINTS

- Immunizations are a cornerstone of the general health of the population.
- Identifying barriers and determining solutions to vaccination obstacles are essential for vaccine uptake.
- Having a skilled and knowledgeable health care team is vital in creating a vaccine-positive practice culture.
- Open dialogue among patients and health care professionals enables effective communication regarding vaccination concerns as well as promoting trust in the provider-patient relationship.
- The single most determinant of vaccine acceptance is a strong recommendation from a health care professional.

INTRODUCTION

Immunizations are a cost-effective public health intervention that averts 2 million to 3 million deaths annually worldwide.[1] Vaccinations continue to be deemed 1 of the 10 greatest public health achievements in the United States by the Centers for Disease Control and Prevention (CDC). Decade after decade, newer vaccines are introduced that continue to lead toward a reduction of health care costs, hospitalizations, and death.[2–4] Through immunization, smallpox has been eradicated, and polio, eliminated in many countries, is on the verge of eradication as well—remaining in Afghanistan, Pakistan, and Nigeria alone.[5]

Vaccines are more widely available now than ever before. Although most individuals continue to be vaccinated in medical offices, there are many locations available for individuals to receive recommended immunizations, including health departments, travel clinics, pharmacies, health care centers, schools, workplaces, and even religious centers/churches. Information about vaccines also is more widely available

Department of Family Medicine, BayCare Medical Group, Palm Harbor, FL, USA
* 3890 Tampa Road, Palm Harbor, Florida, 34684, USA
E-mail address: amraac@gmail.com

Prim Care Clin Office Pract 47 (2020) 395–405
https://doi.org/10.1016/j.pop.2020.05.008
primarycare.theclinics.com

through the Internet from a wide range of sources. Although the physician may continue to be patients' most trusted source of information about immunizations, they are gathering information from a wide variety of sources and may find they have questions and concerns. Intentionally engaging in open dialogue between clinicians, staff, patients, and parents/guardians encourages opportunity for shared decision making and patient autonomy, while allowing opportunities to correct any misinformation or alleviate concerns.

CREATING AND MAINTAINING A VACCINE-POSITIVE CULTURE

The Collaborative Patient Care Team

The foundation of a vaccine-positive culture in clinical practice is a well-trained staff. It is important to educate all clinical and administrative staff regarding the importance of vaccines and the illnesses they prevent.[6] For instance, vaccine-hesitant individuals are more agreeable to immunization when informed *Haemophilus influenzae* and Streptococcus pneumonia are the 2 main causes of meningitis or that a rotavirus infection most likely will lead to a hospital admission and even may result in death.[6] Explaining the significant medical risks from lack of immunization as well as the financial burden incurred from medical bills often depicts a lucid picture regarding the pros and cons of vaccination.[6] **Table 1** provides some examples of possible staff actions in fostering the vaccine culture in the practice.

Table 1
Potential staff roles in a fostering a vaccine-positive culture

Staff Member	Examples of Vaccine Supportive Actions
Appointment scheduler Front desk/ reception	• Reminds patients that vaccines are due when scheduling well visits • Uses supportive language about upcoming vaccines rather than negative language (eg, avoiding "too bad you have to get a shot today") • Assists scheduling well visits at times when immunizations will not be problematic (eg, not the day before the big game or the prom) • Appropriately shares with parents their support of vaccines in their families
Triage/medial assistant	• Prepares patient/family for immunization with encouraging words • Appropriately shares with parents their support of vaccines in their families
Nurse	• Considers patient comfort using pain-relieving techniques • Minimizes discomfort by using efficient technique and preparation • Uses a vaccine information sheet as an opportunity for shared decision making • Answers questions openly and honestly and refers to the clinician when unsure • Appropriately shares with parents support of vaccines in their families
Clinician	• Allows standing orders to support staff in creating a safe but efficient workflow • Leverages huddles to talk about any potential concerns or needs • Shares data about how the practice is doing and where more attention is needed • Appropriately shares with parents support of vaccines in their families • Identifies and supports the vaccine champion

Knowledge and Training

Employees should familiarize themselves with current guidelines and recommendations. In order to do so, they should have access to academic resources, such as the CDC, the American Academy of Pediatrics, and the American Academy of Family Physicians (AAFP).[7] With a strong fund of knowledge, team members should be confident in their role as vaccine advocates.[7] They should have autonomy to identify vaccine-eligible individuals and schedule immunization appointments as well as have standing orders in place to administer vaccines.[7] Use of a standardized system that recognizes patients who need vaccines also is a helpful asset for staff.[8] **Table 2** notes some useful training resources.

Alongside a well-trained staff who are vaccine advocates, designating a "vaccine champion" also is beneficial. This staff member is accountable for vaccine storage, documentation, and administration.[7] Vaccine champions also can collaborate with the physician leader to identify, implement, and sustain practice vaccine delivery improvements; lead, educate, and empower others in a practice; and track key data to report back to the practice. Unlike other practice roles, vaccine champions can be staff members from any area of the practice who has an interest in leading the immunization efforts. Often, they can be recruited from among those who are looking for a leadership opportunity, have an interest in quality improvement, and are willing to dedicate time to immunization work. Many practices allow dedicated paid time for this work, in addition to the title/recognition, and some provide additional compensation. The AAFP developed a practice champion model, which has been used successfully in a variety of behavior change interventions in primary care practices, including immunizations for adults and adolescents. A white paper on the adolescent project is available at https://www.aafp.org/dam/AAFP/documents/patient_care/immunizations/office-champions-final-report.pdf.

Table 2
Immunization training resources for practices

Organization	Web Site	Brief Description
Immunization Action Coalition	www.immunize.org	Variety of resources, including videos, handouts, standing orders, training slide decks, and sample office documentation
AAFP and AAFP Foundation	https://www.aafp.org/patient-care/public-health/immunizations.html https://www.aafp.org/patient-care/public-health/immunizations/vaccines-teens.html	Variety of resources from immunization schedules to white papers, resource libraries, and coding/documentation tools
American Academy of Pediatrics	https://www.aap.org/en-us/advocacy-and-policy/aap-health-initiatives/immunizations/Pages/Immunizations-home.aspx	Variety of resources from immunization schedules to advocacy tools, resource libraries, and coding/documentation tools
Nation HPV Vaccination Roundtable	http://www.hpvroundtable.org/action-guides/	HPV-specific action guides, but most of the tools are useful across vaccines
CDC	https://www.cdc.gov/vaccines/hcp/conversations/index.html	Guide to vaccine conversations with parents with supportive resource tools

Leading by Example

In addition to ensuring patient immunizations are up to date, it also is influential for the clinical staff to be current on their immunizations. This leading by example method illustrates a practice's proimmunization philosophy.[6] A health care office's provaccination policies also can be shared with patients at time of registration and/or clinic visit.[6]

Facilitating Vaccines Through Workflow Design

Prepare for the day by reviewing vaccine status during team huddles. Review standing orders, or pre-order during the huddle, to improve the efficiency of vaccine delivery during rooming. Arrange the practice to allow easy access to vaccine storage as well as a quiet place to review the schedule to confirm orders and prepare the vaccine for delivery. Deliver a strong presumptive recommendation elaborating to explain the need for vaccination as well as its safety and efficacy as needed. This message should be reinforced throughout the visit by all staff, including front office representatives, medical assistants/nursing staff, and medical providers. Encourage shared decision making and create a space open for patient questions. By addressing vaccine concerns at the initial appointment, health care practitioners can improve the uptake rate for future immunizations.[9] Through an open and constant dialogue between staff and patients, a positive and effective vaccine practice culture can be maintained.[6] Use anticipatory guidance to notify patients/parents of upcoming vaccine recommendations.

Identifying and Addressing Barriers to Vaccination

Even in a vaccine-positive environment, there may be barriers to vaccinating that can be a challenge to overcome, including cost, missing work/school, wait times to receive immunization, missed opportunities, anxiety, fear, unpleasant experience/physical pain from vaccination, miseducation/misconception regarding safety and efficacy of vaccines, and vaccine hesitancy.

One major contribution to incomplete or delayed vaccination hinges on socioeconomic factors.[8] Circumstances, such as financial hardship, loss of employment, foreclosure, and/or divorce, can make it difficult to stay abreast of preventive health visits, screenings, and immunizations. In regard to children's vaccines, some parents are single, overworked, and overwhelmed—making it difficult to keep up with their children's vaccinations.[8] In situations where a parent or guardian loses a job and health insurance, the possibility of qualifying for Medicaid is not considered.[8] This, in turn, interrupts continuity of health care.

Coordinating transportation, scheduling time off work, and missing school/daycare also have financial burdens. If caregivers have an hourly job, they are at an economic disadvantage to bringing in children during daytime hours for immunization. For the children who are in daycare, there is no fee deduction for doctors' appointments. Additionally, some facilities do not allow children to return to daycare if they are not in attendance prior to a certain time in the morning or if a certain number of hours are missed in 1 day.

An additional obstacle involves health care facilities that may be difficult to reach, have limited availability/hours, or have significantly long wait times. Some practices give immunizations only by appointment or as part of health supervision (or well child) visits.[10] If a primary care provider does not have the vaccination in stock, waiting to receive immunization creates significant delay and can even result in a missed opportunity for vaccination.

A missed opportunity for vaccination refers to any contact with health services by an individual (child or adult) who is eligible for vaccination (unvaccinated, partially vaccinated, or not up to date and free of contraindications to vaccination), which does not result in the person receiving all the vaccine doses for which the individual is eligible.[11] Several studies have documented that, during approximately half of child health visits, immunizations are due but not given.[12] Missed opportunities contributed 13% of the total under-vaccination time in the suburban practice, 27% in the clinic, and more than 40% in other practices.[13] Another research analysis determined that more than half of preterm infants were under-vaccinated at 19 months, and one-third failed to catch up by 36 months.[14] These missed opportunities result in deficiencies in vaccination status as well as an incomplete immunization record.

A further barrier to vaccination is anxiety regarding needles, fear of receiving injections, and physical pain from vaccination resulting in an unpleasant experience. In 1 study, 24% of parents and 63% of children reported a fear of needles, and needle fear was the primary reason for immunization noncompliance for 7% and 8% of parents and children, respectively.[15] Pain after vaccination and previous unpleasant encounters during immunizations also are notable obstacles. It has been recorded that past experiences with vaccinations and vaccination services, such as negative encounters with vaccine providers, also can influence decision making regarding vaccination.[16,17]

Supplementary to previous negative vaccination visits are concerns regarding the safety and efficacy of immunizations, which further hinder vaccine acceptance (eg, **Box 1**). There is a great deal of misinformation that makes consent to vaccinate difficult. A common issue is the linkage of vaccines with adverse reactions, such as autism, multiple sclerosis, and diabetes.[18] With this preconceived notion, receiving multiple immunizations during a single visit raises further concern about idiopathic chronic diseases, as well as the effects of vaccination on the immune system. Another point of contention is thimerosal—a mercury-containing amalgam used as a preservative to prevent vaccine contamination. Although there was no scientific evidence

Box 1
Common vaccine safety concerns

- Multiple vaccines and their effects on the immune system
- Autism and vaccines
- SIDS
- Febrile seizures after immunization
- Syncope/loss of consciousness/fainting after vaccination
- Thimerosal/mercury content
- Vaccine additives/adjuvants
- Guillain-Barré syndrome
- Immunizations during pregnancy
- Vaccine recalls
- Historical vaccine safety concerns

Adapted from Centers for Disease Control and Prevention. Common vaccine safety concerns. Available at: https://www.cdc.gov/vaccinesafety/concerns/index.html. Accessed September 5, 2019.

behind purported neurotoxic and psychological effects from vaccines containing thimerosal, objection to this compound resulted in swift removal of it from most immunizations (a few flu vaccines still contain thimerosal).[19] Thimerosal and other vaccine adjuvants are prevalent concerns, creating a roadblock to successful vaccination. Although adverse reactions may occur after immunization, it is extremely rare.[20] For example, 1 study noted there was a slightly increased risk of Guillain-Barré syndrome (an uncommon but potential adverse event after influenza vaccination), 8 days to 21 days post-vaccination.[20] Even given the potential increased risk of Guillain-Barré syndrome, however, the benefits of vaccination markedly outweighed the possibility of Guillain-Barré syndrome.[20] Another concern is febrile seizures after immunization. This condition, which affects 3% to 5% of children less than or equal to 6 years old, results in a sudden rise in temperature that precipitates a seizure.[21] Despite a slight correlation between febrile seizures and vaccination, a recent analysis concluded that vaccine-related febrile seizures accounted for a small percentage of all febrile seizure hospitalizations. Furthermore, no difference in outcomes was noted when vaccine-related febrile seizures were compared with non–vaccine-related febrile seizures.[21] Alongside the association of vaccine-related febrile seizures is a matter of syncope after immunization. Nearly all vaccines have been reported to the CDC as a cause of loss of consciousness. The most common includes the human papillomavirus (HPV) vaccine, meningococcal conjugate vaccine, and tetanus/diphtheria/acellular pertussis vaccine after being given to adolescents.[22] Scientists believe fainting is a result of the immunization process and not the vaccine itself, given that the ingredients of all the 3 vaccines are different.[22]

An additional concern is the safety of immunizations in the pregnant and infant population. The influenza virus is highly contagious, and pregnant individuals are among the most vulnerable. Changes in immunity during pregnancy make expectant mothers more susceptible to infections, which may result in further complications, such as preterm labor, hospitalization, miscarriage, and even death. One study noted that although most women knew the flu was highly contagious, approximately 90% incorrectly believed that expectant mothers had the same risk of complications as nonpregnant women.[23] Furthermore, of the women interviewed for the study, only half were aware of flu vaccination recommendations during pregnancy as well as that it was safe during both pregnancy and breastfeeding[23]; 80% of the women surveyed incorrectly assumed that immunization resulted in diseases and birth defects.[23] Contrary to this assumption, a longitudinal analysis determined that a possible linkage between immunization and disorders, such as sudden infant death syndrome (SIDS) and attention-deficit/hyperactivity disorder, were unsupported.[24]

All these concerns lead to another significant barrier to immunization—vaccine hesitancy. As discussed, this broad description encompasses many individuals who

- Refuse some vaccines but are agreeable to other immunizations
- Desire a delayed vaccine schedule
- Are critical of the safety of newer vaccines
- Question relevance/validity of immunization in the modern world
- Lack personal knowledge regarding preventive benefits of vaccines
- Are skeptical due to health professionals'/providers' lack of knowledge and own vaccine hesitancy[16]

In a cross-sectional study, it was concluded if parents perceived a disease as very serious, they were more likely to vaccinate against it.[25] For example, 84% would immunize against meningitis given its increased morbidity and mortality.[25] Only 34%, however, would immunize against chickenpox, believing their child would fully recover from the illness if infected.[25] Some parents desire a delayed vaccination schedule—57% preferred their child receive no more than 2 injections per visit.[25] In addition, more than 50% of parents elected for newer vaccines to be given at a separate visit.[25] Parents are critical regarding the safety of newer immunizations and may focus more on the possible risks of vaccination instead of the dangers from the actual disease the vaccine is preventing.[16] Ironically, immunizations are a victim of their own success. Due to the historical achievements of vaccination, many question the importance of immunizations in today's world. Because of the lack of exposure to diseases that were more prevalent in the past (eg, chickenpox, measles, mumps, rubella, diphtheria, and pertussis), individuals now contemplate how relevant these immunizations are to the current population.[7] Others believe improved hygiene and health care are the reasons why illnesses have declined, and they ponder the validity of vaccines in the modern era.[7] These misconceptions highlight the personal lack of knowledge concerning the preventive benefits of immunization as well as illustrate the perception that severe illnesses/infectious diseases no longer are a threat to the health of the population. In addition to parent/patient vaccine hesitancy is vaccine uncertainty from the health care practitioner. In a study where health care workers were surveyed, 37% felt children received too may immunizations and 36% opined that a healthy way of living could remove the need for vaccination altogether.[16] The reluctance to vaccinate also is exemplified by the considerable amount of health care professionals who avoid immunizations (eg, flu vaccine), even after it is strongly recommended and freely available at their employment site.[16] The lack of awareness from medical professionals, including indications for immunization and contraindications to vaccination, add further to the vaccine hesitancy barrier.

POSSIBLE SOLUTIONS TO BARRIERS

In order to improve vaccination rates, immunization barriers need to be handled astutely. One study determined that increased vaccination rates could be accomplished by improving office practice procedures.[26] In **Box 2**, options for increasing the percentage of vaccinations among both children and adults are listed. Enhancing access to vaccinations is one way to overcome immunization barriers.7 To reduce wait times, health care practices can offer vaccination-only visits. These visits can be made available on a same-day basis and/or during weekend hours. Allowing extended office hours also can make it convenient for patients to receive vaccines. Increasing accessibility also enables individuals to address immunization concerns with their health care team. A well-informed health care provider and staff can make strong recommendations for vaccination. Most people (79%–85%) advised they were more like to accept immunization if their practitioner recommended it.[20] Furthermore, individuals who were doubtful of bureaucratic sources were more willing to trust information from their personal physician who took the time to listen and address their apprehensions regarding vaccine safety.[26]

In order to make a strong recommendation, it is imperative that both the health care provider and staff be well versed in the risks/benefits of vaccination, current immunization guidelines, and data backing the prevention of diseases through vaccination. It also is vital that a health care team be able to address any concerns or hesitancy one may have regarding vaccination. An effective tool for this is Singer's C.A.S.E. method (**Fig. 1**), which is a 4-step model that integrates fact-based guidance with an empathy-based educational approach.[27] Through this strategy, an individual's vaccination concerns are recognized and a commonality is identified.[28] By corroboration, the health care professional discusses expertise on vaccines, explains the science behind

Box 2
Recommendations for vaccine promotion

Accessibility
- Availability of same-day/walk-in appointments for vaccinations.
- Allow nurse visits for immunizations.
- Reduce office wait times.
- Extend office hours/offer weekend appointments.
- Permit visits for vaccine-hesitant patients/parents to discuss concerns.
- Have a supportive and educated staff.

Provider/staff education
- Be informed about vaccines and current guidelines for immunization.
- Explain data/research regarding vaccines.
- Recount the illnesses vaccines prevent.
- Detail the possible health and financial implications of vaccine noncompliance.
- Address patient/parent concerns.
- Distribute educational materials.
- Provider should make strong recommendations.

Optimization of patient visits
- Issue a vaccination record at visit and provide immunizations that are due.
- Administer eligible vaccines at acute, follow-up, and annual wellness visits.
- Have standing orders in place to provide vaccines.
- Offer combination vaccines.

Resource utilization
- Provide reminders when vaccinations are due.
- Use electronic medal records for setting immunization alerts
- Employ vaccine registry to determine vaccine eligible patients.
- Vaccine ambassadors for vaccine-hesitant parents
- Promote vaccination.
- Internal audit of immunization rates in practice and of individual providers

Data from Refs.[6,26,30]

immunization, and subsequently gives advice based on that science.[28] This creates an open environment for positive communication between patients/parents and health care providers. Alongside an open line of communication, educational materials, such as vaccine information sheets, can be provided for further information.

In addition to improving patient access and increasing health care professionals' knowledge, opportunities for immunization need to be identified and available resources need to be maximized. For instance, patients who are due for vaccines can be immunized at their follow-up or sick visits—not just at their annual wellness appointment. Studies have exhibited that vaccinating patients at acute visits may decrease their subsequent need for medical care.[6]

Immunizations also can be a category of a patient's medical history (similar to past medical history, family history, social history, and so forth), where it is updated at each visit and the patient is notified of when the next vaccination is due. Also, by offering combination vaccines and having standing orders in place for immunization, vaccine compliance improves and the need for a return visit minimized. For example, in 1 study, 63% of patients were more likely to receive immunization if a standing order was in place compared with only 38% willing to receive vaccination without a standing order program.[29] Additionally, incorporating alerts in the electronic medical records, as well as making use of a vaccine registry, helps identify vaccine eligible patients. These systems also are great resources in providing patient reminders as to when they are due for immunizations.

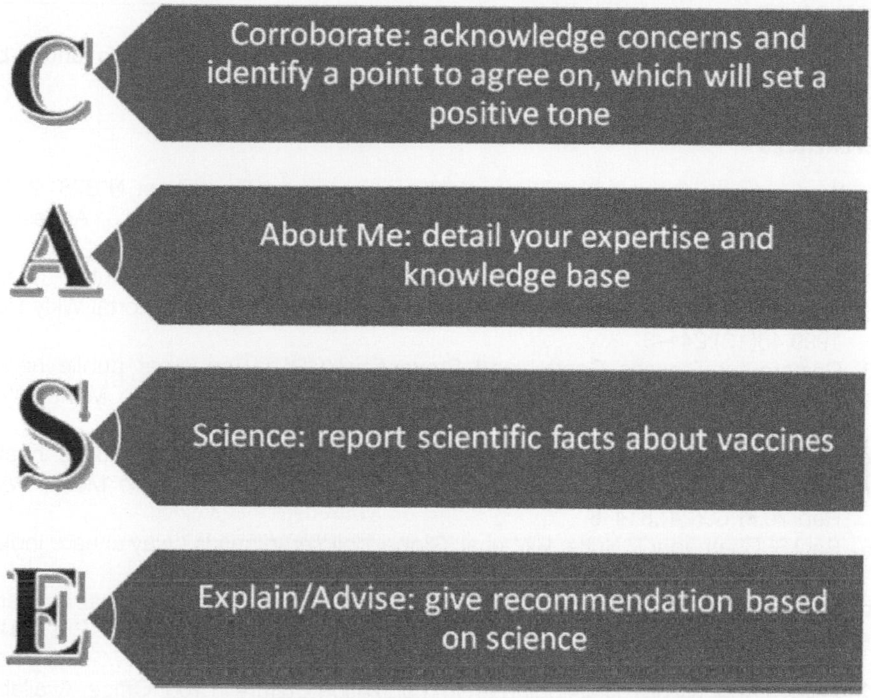

Fig. 1. C.A.S.E. method. (*Adapted from* Singer A. Communicating vaccine safety information to parents: a new framework Available at: https://cdc.confex.com/cdc/nic2010/webprogram/Paper22643.html. Accessed September 26, 2019; with permission.)

A novel approach is health care practitioners identifying their patients who are vaccine ambassadors—individuals who are willing to receive vaccine training and share their reasons for immunization with vaccine-hesitant patients.[30] One study determined that vaccine hesitancy decreased from 23% to 14%.[30] Additionally, the number of individuals who agreed vaccination was beneficial increased.[30] Further vaccine promotion can be done through vaccine reminders/mailers, social media publicity, and informational items available on office bulletin boards. In 1 study, a completion rate for a 3-dose vaccine was reported to be approximately 10% higher for a group who had received a reminder when compared with a control group.[6] Internal practice audits also can be helpful in achieving increased vaccination rates. A systematic literature review noted that though practice audit and feedback, immunization rates may improve up to 49%.[31]

SUMMARY

Without question, immunizations have decreased, and even eradicated, infectious diseases. Vaccination is the best way to protect oneself as well as the general population from threatening diseases across the life span. Although barriers to vaccination continue to exist, it is possible to implement methods as a solution to these barriers. Accessibility to receive vaccinations, knowledgeable health care professionals, optimized patient visits, and appropriate utilization of resources have a positive impact on vaccination rates and support establishing a vaccine-positive culture.

DISCLOSURE

2017 Graduate of the AAFP Vaccine Science Fellowship. The fellowship is funded by an unrestricted grant from Merck Sharp & Dohme Corporation.

REFERENCES

1. World Health Organization. Immunization coverage - Fact sheet N°378. 2015. Available at: http://who.int/mediacentre/factsheets/fs378/en/. Accessed November 19, 2019.
2. Centers for Disease Control and Prevention (CDC). Ten great public health achievements – United States, 1900-1999, 1999. MMWR Morb Mortal Wkly Rep 1999;48(12):241–3.
3. Centers for Disease Control and Prevention (CDC). Ten great public health achievements — United States, 2001—2010, 2010. MMWR Morb Mortal Wkly Rep 2010;60(19):619–23.
4. Centers for Disease Control and Prevention (CDC). Ten great public health achievements — United States, 2001—2010, 2011. MMWR Morb Mortal Wkly Rep 2011;60(24):814–8.
5. Bahl S, Bhatnagar P, Sutter RW, et al. Global polio eradication - way ahead. Indian J Pediatr 2018;85(2):124–31.
6. Ventola CL. Immunization in the United States: recommendations, barriers, and measures to improve compliance: part 1: childhood vaccinations. P T 2016; 41(7):426–36.
7. Give2menacwy.org. Developing an Immunization Culture in Your Office. Available at: https://www.give2menacwy.org/pdfs/immunization-culture.pdf. Accessed August 1, 2019.
8. Temoka E. Becoming a vaccine champion: evidence-based interventions to address the challenges of vaccination. S D Med 2013;(Spec no):68–72.
9. Holt D, Bouder F, Elemuwa C, et al. The importance of the patient voice in vaccination and vaccine safety—are we listening? Clin Microbiol Infect 2016;22: S146–53.
10. Institute of Medicine (US). Committee on Overcoming Barriers to Immunization. In: Durch JS, editor. Overcoming barriers to immunization: a Workshop summary. Washington, DC: National Academies Press (US); 1994. p. 2. Immunization and the Health Care System. Available at: https://www.ncbi.nlm.nih.gov/books/NBK231201/. Accessed September 2, 2019.
11. Magadzire BP, Joao G, Shendale S, et al. Reducing missed opportunities for vaccination in selected provinces of Mozambique: A study protocol. Gates Open Res 2017;1:5.
12. Wood D, Schuster M, Donald-Sherbourne C, et al. Reducing missed opportunities to vaccinate during child health visits: how effective are parent education and case management? Arch Pediatr Adolesc Med 1998;152(3):238–43.
13. Szilagyi PG, Rodewald LE, Humiston SG, et al. Missed opportunities for childhood vaccinations in office practices and the effect on vaccination status. Pediatrics 1993;91(1):1–7.
14. Hofstetter AM, Jacobson EN, Dehart MP, et al. Early childhood vaccination status of preterm infants. Pediatrics 2019;144(3). https://doi.org/10.1542/peds.2018-3520.
15. Taddio A, Ipp M, Thivakaran S, et al. Survey of the prevalence of immunization non-compliance due to needle fears in children and adults. Vaccine 2012;30: 4807–12.

16. Dubé E, Laberge C, Guay M, et al. Vaccine hesitancy: an overview. Hum Vaccin Immunother 2013;9(8):1763–73.
17. CDC. Centers for Disease Control and Prevention. Common Vaccine Safety Concerns. In: Vaccine Safety. 2016. Available at: https://www.cdc.gov/vaccinesafety/concerns/index.html. Accessed September 5, 2019.
18. Zimmerman RK, Wolfe RM, Fox DE, et al. Vaccine criticism on the World Wide Web. J Med Internet Res 2005;7(2):e17.
19. Offit PA. Thimerosal and vaccines – a cautionary tale. N Engl J Med 2007;357(13):1278–9.
20. Perez-Vilar S, Wernecke M, Arya D, et al. Surveillance for Guillain-Barré syndrome after influenza vaccination among U.S. Medicare beneficiaries during the 2017–2018 season. Vaccine 2019;37(29):3856–65.
21. Deng L, Gidding H, Macartney K, et al. Postvaccination Febrile seizure severity and outcome. Pediatrics 2019;143(5). https://doi.org/10.1542/peds.2018-2120.
22. CDC. Centers for Disease Control and Prevention. Fainting (Syncope) Concerns. In: Vaccine Safety. 2016. Available at: https://www.cdc.gov/vaccinesafety/concerns/fainting.html. Accessed September 9, 2019.
23. Yudin MH, Salaripour M, Sgro MD. Pregnant women's knowledge of influenza and the use and safety of the influenza vaccine during pregnancy. J Obstet Gynaecol Can 2009;31(2):120–5.
24. Yang YT, Shaw J. Sudden infant death syndrome, attention-deficit/hyperactivity disorder and vaccines: Longitudinal population analyses. Vaccine 2018;36(5):595–8.
25. Bedford H, Lansley M. More vaccines for children? Parents' views. Vaccine 2007;25(45):7818–23.
26. Anderson EL. Recommended solutions to the barriers to immunization in children and adults. Mo Med 2014;111(4):344–8.
27. Hagood EA, Mintzer Herlihy S. Addressing heterogeneous parental concerns about vaccination with a multiple-source model: a parent and educator perspective. Hum Vaccin Immunother 2013;9(8):1790–4.
28. Singer A. Communicating vaccine safety information to parents: a new framework. Available at: https://cdc.confex.com/cdc/nic2010/webprogram/Paper22643.html. Accessed September 26, 2019.
29. Goebel L, Neitch S, Mufson M. Standing orders in an ambulatory setting increases influenza vaccine usage in older people. J Am Geriatr Soc 2005;53(6):1008–10.
30. Smith TC. Vaccine rejection and hesitancy: a review and call to action. Open Forum Infect Dis 2017;4(3):ofx146.
31. Bordley W, Chelminski A, Margolis P, et al. The effect of audit and feedback on immunization delivery. Am J Prev Med 2000;18(4):343–50.

Creating a Sustainable Vaccine Delivery Practice

Jamie Loehr, MD

KEYWORDS

• Vaccine delivery practice • Vaccine logistics • Vaccine billing

KEY POINTS

- Setting up an effective and financially viable vaccine delivery practice is a team effort requiring a vaccine champion, vaccine coordinators, and support from the entire office staff.
- There are several best-practice recommendations available whether the practice is starting from scratch or seeking to improve the current process in the office.
- Vaccine delivery involves appropriate storing and monitoring of the vaccines, meticulous administration of the immunization to patients, and accurate documentation.
- Appropriate billing for vaccine administration can provide a steady income to the office even as patients receive necessary preventive care.

Most organizations realize that providing vaccines to patients is good medical care. By offering the vaccine in the office, there is no delay in protection against the disease. In contrast, if a patient needs to go elsewhere to receive the vaccine, that simple barrier delays the protection, sometimes forever. There are data that when pregnant patients defer flu vaccines at a given visit, only about 50% of them receive the flu vaccine later in the season.[1]

However, the process of providing vaccines places a significant logistical burden on the practice, and to do it in a financially viable manner is even more difficult. The goal of this article is to facilitate the process for any organization, large or small, whether the practice is starting from scratch or is looking to improve the process in its office.

For more detailed guidelines on best practices with vaccine delivery, please refer to the US Centers for Disease Control and Prevention (CDC) Vaccine Storage and Handling Toolkit (www.cdc.gov/vaccines/hcp/admin/storage/toolkit/storage-handling-toolkit.pdf) and the Immunization Action Coalition's document: Vaccinating Adults: A Step-by-Step Guide (www.immunize.org/guide/).

Cayuga Family Medicine, 302 West Seneca Street, Ithaca, NY 14850, USA
E-mail address: Dr.Jamie.Loehr@Gmail.com

Prim Care Clin Office Pract 47 (2020) 407–418
https://doi.org/10.1016/j.pop.2020.05.009

CREATING A TEAM

Office Staff

The first step is generating enough will in the organization to add, or expand, vaccine delivery as a service. This step may simple in a small two-physician office but is more complicated if the facility is larger. Adding this service line requires buy-in from clinical and financial leaders in the practice. They must believe in the mission and be willing to support it with enough resources to make it successful.

In addition, the frontline staff will be directly affected. The front office staff will need to make more appointments, the nurses will need to give the vaccines and do the documentation, and the billing staff need to be prepared for the extra work and complexity of billing for vaccines. It helps if all the staff recognize the vital importance of providing vaccines to patients in the office as well as the benefits to the patients, the community, and the practice.

Vaccine Champion

One best practice is to have a vaccine champion in the office. This person is the advocate for the vaccines, the one who reminds everyone why they vaccinate and helps push the project forward. A champion should also be aware of the policy issues around vaccines, and keep up to date on new recommendations from the Advisory Committee on Immunization Practices and the CDC.

Vaccine Coordinator

Note that the vaccine champion is not necessarily the vaccine coordinator, although, in a small office, one person might share the role. A vaccine coordinator is the logistical expert of the vaccination process. The coordinator's role is to make sure everything runs smoothly. The responsibilities might include ordering and installing equipment; ordering the vaccines and other necessary supplies, such as needles and syringes; writing protocols, such as how to give and document vaccines; writing policies on standing orders; and, if appropriate, reporting vaccines to the immunization registry. In addition, each coordinator needs a backup coordinator to fill in when the primary person is unavailable.

Providing vaccines in an office is a team effort. Like so much else in medicine, the team performs at a higher level than the individual. For example, the front staff can tell the patient at check in that the flu vaccine is now available, the nurse can offer the vaccine to the patient, and, if there is a standing order, even give the vaccine before the physician enters the room. By using everyone in the office as an advocate for vaccines, it is much more likely that the patient will leave the visit having received the necessary vaccines for that day.

STRUCTURE AND SPACE

Storage Units

The first question to ask when providing vaccines in the office is where they are going to be stored. Most vaccines require refrigeration and the remaining few require a freezer. The current storage guidelines recommend separate units; specifically, a dedicated refrigerator and a dedicated freezer.

Although a combination refrigerator/freezer unit can be used, it should not be used to store vaccines in the freezer because there are more temperature fluctuations in a combination unit. A small dormitory or bar refrigerator also has temperature fluctuations and should never be used.

Work Space

In addition to the physical space for the refrigerator and freezer, the vaccine coordinator should set up a work space for preparing the vaccines. The work space should be close to the storage units so staff do not need to walk far with the vaccines. It should also offer some privacy. Working with vaccines is a meticulous process and too much distraction can interfere with accurately preparing and documenting the vaccines.

All the supplies needed for the vaccines should be readily accessible at the workstation, including syringes, needles, gauze, alcohol wipes, Band-Aids, and labels. Labels are useful when staff are drawing up vaccines into a plain syringe and need to remember which vaccine is in which syringe. In addition, the work space needs easy access to a sharps container in case needles need to be disposed of while working.

TEMPERATURE MONITORING

The goal of proper vaccine storage is to preserve the cold chain, a guarantee that the vaccine stays at an appropriate temperature. If a vaccine is exposed to temperatures out of range for a prolonged period of time, the vaccine may be rendered less potent or even useless. This situation can lead to significant wastage and, in a worst-case scenario, the dose may even need to be repeated.

The required temperature range for the refrigerator is 2°C to 8°C (36°F–46° F) whereas for the freezer it is less than −15°C (5° F). Those temperatures should be prominently displayed on the unit for easy reference. Make sure that the refrigerator and freezer have had time to stabilize their temperatures before storing any vaccines; this may take several days.

Current best practices recommend that each unit has a dedicated 24-hour temperature monitor with an alarm. The days of only recording the temperature with a written log are long gone. The monitor should record the temperature at least every 30 minutes.

The monitor is usually kept outside the storage unit, whereas the probe inside is connected either wirelessly or via a wired connection that slips in at the edge of the door. Using a buffered temperature probe is also recommended because that prevents erratic temperature excursions from merely opening and closing the door.

Another best practice is for the temperature monitor to be officially calibrated and to have a certificate of calibration. Temperature monitors can drift over time and become less accurate. Thus, the calibration should be repeated, often every 1 to 2 years, based on the manufacturer's recommendations.

Remote Alarm System

Another consideration in placing the storage units in the office is remote access to the alarm system. Although it helps to know that the alarm went off over the weekend, so that spoiled vaccines are not used, it is best if someone is informed immediately if there is a temperature excursion. The vaccine coordinator then has the opportunity to intervene immediately and possibly save the vaccines from spoilage.

Although some temperature monitors have a built-in alarm system that informs someone on the staff remotely of any problems, many times the practice has to buy a separate remote alarm system. This system can call the vaccine coordinator or send a text or email message when the alarm goes off. Whichever system a practice uses, it is necessary to provide access to a phone line and/or the Internet. This requirement is often difficult if the practice is retrofitting an existing space and it needs to be considered in the planning.

Power Supply

In addition, the importance of reliable electricity is paramount. The vaccine coordinator must make sure the power outlet can handle the required loads of the storage units. In addition, the outlets and power cords should be clearly marked with signs that say "Do Not Unplug". A safety-lock plug or an outlet cover that prevents accidental unplugging is a good idea. There should be a similar warning sign at the circuit breaker so that no one turns off the power accidently. Sample signs are available at the Immunization Action Coalition Web site: https://www.immunize.org/catg.d/p2090.pdf and https://www.immunize.org/catg.d/p2091.pdf.

PAPERWORK

Temperature Logs

Although handwritten temperature logs are no longer recommended as the sole method of documenting temperatures, they still have their place in the vaccine monitoring process. Although the continuous data can be downloaded and saved weekly, a daily log requires someone to check the temperature and document it at least twice a day. This checking is useful if the monitoring system does not have an audible alarm. Some monitors only have a visual alarm and every practice needs a system to check that on a regular basis.

Inventory

Managing inventory is a critical function of the vaccine coordinator. The numbers are usually kept on a computer spreadsheet to be able to show trends over time. Although ordering vaccines is discussed later, keeping track of the supply ensures that enough vaccine is available when a patient is in the office. It is frustrating (and embarrassing) to have a patient arrive for a scheduled vaccine visit and not have the vaccine in the refrigerator. Most offices manage inventory manually with a full count each week. While doing this, be careful of the temperature in the storage unit because repeatedly opening and closing the refrigerator risks sending the temperature out of range.

Vaccine Information Sheets

Vaccine information sheets [VISs] are documents that summarize each vaccine in a succinct two-page handout. They are produced by the CDC and go over the risks and benefits of each vaccine, including specific contraindications when a vaccine should not be given. It is a federal requirement to hand out the VIS to each patient or parent before the immunization.

There are many ways to give a VIS. The most common choice is a paper copy, partly because the patient/parent needs the option to carry the information out of the office after the appointment. However, the patient may decline the paper copy and read the information in other ways. Some offices have a laminated VIS for patients to read, others present the VIS on the computer screen in the room, and patients can also download the VIS on their phones or other mobile devices.

VIS files can be downloaded from the CDC or the Immunization Action Coalition web site. Each VIS has a publication date and it is important to keep up to date with the most recent VIS. A list of publication dates is available at www.immunize.org/vis/. In addition, VISs have been translated and are currently available in more than 40 languages.

POLICIES

Each office must understand the laws governing vaccine practices in its own state. Laws vary widely across state lines. For example, in many states, medical assistants are allowed to administer vaccines, whereas in other states, only licensed practical nurses or registered nurses (RNs) can give injections. In some states, unlicensed personnel can be appropriately trained and allowed to administer immunizations. In these states, a trained front office staff person can do double duty and also give vaccines to patients.

Standing Orders

State laws also vary with regard to standing orders. Standing orders are policies that allow a vaccine to be administered to a patient based on a written protocol instead of an individual patient order. In effect, it delegates the decision to give a vaccine to a patient. However, the ultimate responsibility is still with the physician who signed the standing order. The most common use for standing orders is during a flu clinic where dozens or hundreds of patients receive the flu vaccine in a day.

Standing orders have been clearly shown to improve vaccination rates. More than 30 studies across a wide range of practice environments have shown that about 20% more people get vaccinated with standing orders.[2] However, they need to be set up correctly to be effective.

First, state laws need to be respected. In some states, only RNs can implement standing orders, whereas other states are more flexible. Next, the order needs to be clear about the who, what, and when of the vaccine. Who is eligible for a given vaccine? Is it age based (anyone >65 years of age) or disease based (anyone without a functioning spleen)? Which vaccine is allowed? There are several different types of flu vaccines and some are not recommended for given disease states. In addition, when is the vaccine to be given and how often? The flu vaccine is given yearly, whereas other vaccines are only given once.

The good news is that much of this work has already been done. The Immunization Action Coalition has a set of standard orders for adults and children that vaccine coordinators can use as a starting point and modify for their offices. These documents are available at https://www.immunize.org/standing-orders/

ORDERING VACCINES

After everything has been put in place, the office is ready to order vaccines. For some offices, the vaccine coordinator is able to order from a parent organization such as a university or central office. This ability can simplify the decision process because the decisions about which brand to order are made by the parent organization.

However, other offices have to order vaccines for themselves. This process varies by state and also depends on whether the patient is an adult or a child.

Vaccines for Children

If the practice vaccinates children, it should consider participating in the Vaccines for Children (VFC) program. This program is federally funded and provides vaccines free of charge to children whose families might otherwise be unable to afford the vaccine. The rules for which children are eligible for VFC vaccines vary by state but more than one-third of children across the country receive their vaccines through VFC.[3] If the practice does not participate in VFC, those children will have to receive vaccines outside of the office, which might lead to missed opportunities.

Some states have a similar vaccine program for adults who are underinsured or uninsured. In addition, some states are universal purchase states where the state buys all vaccines for all children, including children who have private insurance.

For these programs mentioned earlier, the vaccine coordinator orders the vaccines from the VFC program or the state and does not have to buy them for the practice.

Independently Ordering Vaccines

However, depending on the situation, the practice might need to order vaccines for privately insured patients. This process requires a bit of effort to find the best combination of price and convenience.[4]

There are several vaccine purchasing groups that practices can sign up with, often through their local or state medical societies. They are able to obtain discounts because of bulk purchasing and can usually have the vaccine shipped directly to the office. Another advantage is just having one location for making all the purchases across multiple vaccine manufacturers.

Alternatively, the vaccine coordinator can often buy vaccines from a medical supply company, the one that sells the practice other supplies such as needles and Band-Aids. In general, their prices are higher than can be found elsewhere but that might be worth it for the convenience.

Buying Directly from the Manufacturer

A different option is buying directly from the manufacturer. The vaccine coordinator simply creates an account and starts ordering vaccines. This approach is less convenient because the practice has to maintain accounts with each manufacturer, but the pricing is excellent and usually comes with a small prompt-payment discount. In addition, different manufacturers provide loyalty discounts that rival those of the vaccine purchasing groups.

In addition, the manufacturers usually offer the practice a 60-day to 90-day payment schedule that allows it to defer the payment but still maintain the prompt payment discount. This option allows the practice to start recouping the cost of the vaccine before the payment is due.

When ordering, remember to take the timing of the delivery into account in order to maintain the inventory. Although vaccines are usually delivered from the manufacturer in 2 business days, other organizations, such as VFC, are often not as prompt. In addition, there might be specific rules about how often the practice can order vaccines. For example, 1 state program for underinsured and uninsured adults only allows providers to order vaccines once a year because of an inconsistent funding stream.

MANAGING VACCINE DELIVERIES

Accepting vaccine deliveries requires meticulous attention to detail. First, the staff must make sure that the package is immediately delivered to the vaccine coordinator. If a package sits too long with the deliveries of office supplies, the cold chain might be broken and the integrity of the vaccines might be compromised.

Inspect

Next, the vaccines should be inspected to ensure there was no damage along the way. Also check the cold chain monitor device to make sure there was no temperature excursion during transport. This monitor is an object that changes color when out of temperature range for too long. In addition, check the contents against the packing list and confirm that the expiration dates have not passed.

After inspection, store the vaccines in the appropriate refrigerator or freezer and update the inventory. If the practice is receiving vaccines from different programs, the staff should mark the vaccine so that they know which vaccine belongs to which program. This process might be easier if the practice keeps the vaccines from one program, say VFC, in a different refrigerator, but small offices might not have the option of having a separate unit for each program.

Storage Suggestions

When placing the vaccines in the unit, organize the vaccines so that the vaccines with the earliest expiration dates are toward the front. This process avoids having expired vaccines in the inventory.

The staff should also make sure the unit is not too crowded with vaccines, because that can affect temperature regulation. However, fill any empty space with material that will stabilize temperatures. Water bottles are a good choice to use in the doors of the refrigerator but using some of the cold packing material that comes in the delivery package is also acceptable.

Managing Diluent

One final note: some vaccines come with a specific diluent. This diluent is combined with dried vaccine to prepare the final injection. A common error in vaccine delivery is to just give the diluent without mixing it with the dried vaccine. This error is understandable because most vaccines come in one vial with a liquid, and just grabbing the liquid vial is similar to what the staff does the rest of the time.

To avoid this problem, consider taking an extra step when vaccines with diluents arrive. If the diluent is also kept in the refrigerator (and some diluents are not, being stored at room temperature), tape the diluent and the vaccine together in a bundle of two vials. Then, when the staff reach for that vaccine, they pull both vials out at the same time, minimizing the chance for errors.

VACCINE ADMINISTRATION

The most important thing to remember about vaccine administration is that human beings make mistakes. The goal is to set up checks and balances to try to minimize the number of mistakes and catch them before they affect the patients.

The first step in the process is ordering the vaccine, which means that this provider would like to administer a certain vaccine to a certain patient. This step could be a standing order, an electronic order in the electronic medical record, or circling a vaccine name on a piece of paper.

Avoiding Mistakes

However, staff members receiving these orders should not blindly accept them as correct. They should use their training, knowledge, and office protocols to catch any mistakes. Did the physician order DTaP for a 7-year-old patient instead of the recommended Tdap? Is this vaccine being ordered too early or too late according to the schedule? Is there any chance the patient is pregnant and needs a pregnancy test before receiving the measles, mumps, and rubella (MMR) or varicella vaccine? Each member of the team needs to feel comfortable speaking up if something seems incorrect.

Along similar lines, everyone should speak up if there is a financial issue at stake. Some insurances do not cover certain vaccines and patients need to know whether they are going to be financially responsible. They might choose to get the vaccine elsewhere or defer the vaccine until the insurance question is resolved.

Remember that all patients need a VIS when receiving a vaccine. All too often this is given at the same time (or even after) the vaccine is given. If the staff can give the VIS while the vaccine is being prepared, it gives the patient the needed time to review the VIS without being rushed.

The next step is choosing the vaccines. If there are multiple sources of vaccines (VFC vs private supply), the staff needs to make sure the vaccine comes from the correct supply. They then need to check the expiration date. Even though expiration dates should be monitored during the inventory process, mistakes happen and this is a double check on the process.

When preparing the vaccines, the staff should be in a quiet work space to avoid distractions. The vaccines need to be drawn up safely and properly labeled if drawn up into a separate syringe. Appropriate supplies should be added to the tray and a safe transport method (if needed) arranged to get the vaccines to the patient.

Double Check

Although not required, a double-check system provides backup in making sure that the person who originally drew up the vaccine did not make a mistake. The second person checks to make sure the vaccine drawn up matches the vaccine ordered, that the vaccine is not expired, and that the vaccine is appropriate for the patient. Although much of medicine is digitalized and some systems even use bar codes for tracking, a paper system can work just as well here.

When giving the vaccines, the staff should check the name and date of birth of the patient to avoid any confusion. It also helps if the staff announces the vaccines that are about to be administered. This measure is a final check so the patient can intervene if the wrong vaccine is about to be given. For specific details on how to administer vaccines, please refer to the Immunization Action Coalition Web site (https://www.immunize.org/handouts/administering-vaccines.asp). The staff can also review a video prepared by the California Department of Public Health at https://www.youtube.com/watch?v=WsZ6NEijlfI&t=12s.

EMERGENCY PREPAREDNESS

All offices need an emergency action plan in case of a severe reaction to a vaccine.[5] Anaphylaxis occurs 1 or 2 times for every million doses. Generalized symptoms such as respiratory distress or hypotension can be life threatening and require immediate treatment with epinephrine while waiting for emergency medical services to arrive. Every office should have at least 3 doses of epinephrine available and have regular training in how to manage this situation. More information and standing orders on how to manage adverse reactions can be found at https://www.immunize.org/catg.d/p3082.pdf for adults and https://www.immunize.org/catg.d/p3082a.pdf for children.

Milder reactions, such as itching or simple localized swelling, can be managed with cold compresses and diphenhydramine. However, if the staff have any concerns, they should monitor these patients for 15 to 30 minutes to make sure they do not progress to generalized symptoms.

Some patients have vasovagal reactions after receiving a vaccine and get lightheaded or dizzy, and some people even faint, especially adolescents and young adults. The human papilloma virus vaccine has a specific recommendation that patients be monitored for 15 minutes after receiving the injection. Some providers recommend that all adolescents be observed for 15 minutes after a vaccination in order to minimize any injury should they faint.[4] Of note, 80% of fainting episodes occur in the first 15 minutes after vaccine injection.

In addition, any significant health concern that might be linked to a vaccine needs to be reported to the Vaccine Adverse Event Reporting System (VAERS). VAERS is a vaccine surveillance system jointly run by the CDC and the US Food and Drug Administration. Anyone with a concern can make a report to VAERS, including medical staff, vaccine manufacturers, and even patients or the general public. The person reporting the concern does not have to be sure that the event was related to a vaccine in order to report it.

DOCUMENTATION

After administering a vaccine, certain information is required to be documented under federal law. Specifically, with each vaccination, the staff should document the following:

The name of the vaccine and manufacturer
The date of administration
The lot number
The expiration date
How the vaccine was administered (oral, intramuscular, subcutaneous)
Where in the body the vaccine was administered
Who administered the vaccine
The date of publication of the VIS given to the patient
The date the VIS was given to the patient

The staff should also document any adverse reaction noted in the office. In addition, each patient should have easy access to proof of which vaccines were given. This proof can be a vaccine card, a printout of the vaccines that were given, or electronic access to the vaccine record.

BILLING

In general, there are two components to discuss when talking about billing for vaccines: the charge for the cost of the vaccine and the administration charge.[5]

If the practice received vaccines free as part of a state or federal program (eg, VFC or a state universal purchase vaccine plan), it obviously cannot charge for the cost of the vaccine because the practice did not pay for it. However, it can usually still bill for the administration fee. The billing staff would need to review the details of the particular program in the state to clarify the options.

Billing the Cost of the Vaccine

However, if the practice is billing for vaccines that it purchased privately, it is supposed to bill for the cost of the vaccine. The practice should know that different insurances reimburse for the same vaccine at different rates and that these rates can vary widely. It would be worthwhile for the billing staff to keep track of the various rates so that the practice is reimbursed fairly.

The billing staff should also know that sometimes the insurance reimbursement rate is less than the price the practice paid for the vaccine. Thus, with that insurance, the practice is losing money with each vaccine given. In this situation, the billing staff can take some actual invoices and present them to the insurance company and ask them to adjust their rates. This option sometimes works.

However, the vaccine coordinator can also use this information to seek out a lower-cost source of the vaccine. Some insurance companies peg the reimbursement rate at slightly more than the lowest price of the vaccine available on the market. Therefore, if the practice is being reimbursed too little, it might mean that it is paying too much for the vaccine.

Billing Vaccine Administration Codes

One critical detail to understand is that pediatric vaccine administration codes are different than adult administration codes. Specifically, if a provider, such as a doctor of medicine, nurse practitioner, or physician assistant, provides counseling to a patient or parent on the day of the vaccine administration for a patient less than 19 years of age, the practice is allowed to use Current Procedural Terminology (CPT) codes 90460 and 90461, the pediatric administration codes. Note that, under these guidelines, an 18-year-old patient is still considered eligible for pediatric codes.

However, if a provider does not provide counseling or if the patient is aged 19 years or older, the billing staff should use the adult vaccine administration codes 90471 and 90472. Of note, there are also a few special vaccine administration codes for patients with Medicare, such as G0008 for the influenza vaccine.

The key distinction between the pediatric and adult codes is that the practice is allowed to bill by component for pediatric codes but by vaccine for adult codes. An influenza vaccine only has one component but the MMR vaccine and the Tdap vaccine each have three components. Some pediatric combination vaccines have five components.

Pediatric Billing Code Example

To see an example of how this works in real life, imagine a 5-year-old well visit where the practice gives the MMR-V (MMR and varicella) vaccine and the DTaP-IPV (DTaP

Table 1
Pediatric billing code examples

Vaccine	Admin Code	Reimbursement ($)
Without Counseling		
MMR-V	90471	50
DTaP-Polio	90472	25
—	—	Total: 75
With Counseling		
MMR-V		
First component	90460	50
Second component	90461	25
Third component	90461	25
Fourth component	90461	25
DTaP-Polio		
First component	90460	50
Second component	90461	25
Third component	90461	25
Fourth component	90461	25
—	—	Total: 250

Abbreviations: DTaP, diphtheria, tetanus, and pertussis; MMR-V, measles, mumps, rubella, and varicella.

and polio) vaccine. Without counseling, the practice is allowed to bill for each vaccine. The first vaccine administration code is 90471 and might pay $50, and each subsequent vaccine administration on the same day is 90472 which might pay $25. The total for administering the two vaccines is $75.

However, with counseling, the practice is allowed to bill for each component. For each four-component vaccine, the billing staff can bill 90460 for the first component and 90461 for each of the three additional components. If the 90460 pays the same $50 and the 90461 $25, the practice earns $50 × 2 plus $25 × 6 for a total of $250.00 for administering both vaccines (**Table 1**).

Thus, by adding medically appropriate counseling to the pediatric patients, the practice can receive $250.00 instead of $75 for administering two vaccines,[4] and this does not include billing for the cost of the vaccines.

This is clearly a function of combination vaccines. The benefits do not add up so dramatically with single-component vaccines. However, even there, if the staff administers two single-component vaccines to a child with counseling, the practice will earn more because two 90460s pay more than a 90471 and a 90472.

Box 1
Key resources

Implementing a vaccine delivery program
- Immunization Action Coalition: Vaccinating Adults: A Step-by-Step Guide: www.immunize.org/guide/

Vaccine storage and handling
- CDC toolkit: www.cdc.gov/vaccines/hcp/admin/storage/toolkit/storage-handling-toolkit.pdf

General best-practice guidelines for immunization
- www.cdc.gov/vaccines/hcp/acip-recs/general-recs/downloads/general-recs.pdf

Warning signs: vaccines and power supply
- Wall outlet: www.immunize.org/catg.d/p2090.pdf
- Circuit breaker: www.immunize.org/catg.d/p2091.pdf

Vaccine information sheets
- www.immunize.org/vis/

Standing orders
- www.immunize.org/standing-orders/

Managing adverse reactions
- General: www.cdc.gov/vaccines/hcp/acip-recs/general-recs/downloads/general-recs.pdf, page 72
- Adults: www.immunize.org/catg.d/p3082.pdf
  - Table 5-2: www.cdc.gov/vaccines/hcp/acip-recs/general-recs/downloads/general-recs.pdf
- Children: www.immunize.org/catg.d/p3082a.pdf
  - Table 5-1: www.cdc.gov/vaccines/hcp/acip-recs/general-recs/downloads/general-recs.pd

Vaccine billing tools
- Loehr J. Immunizations: How to Protect Patients and the Bottom Line. Fam Pract Manag. 2015 Mar-Apr;22(2):24–29, www.aafp.org/fpm/2015/0300/p24.html
- American Academy of Family Physicians Resources: https://www.aafp.org/practice-management/payment/coding/admin.html
- American Academy of Pediatric Resources: www.aap.org/en-us/professional-resources/practice-transformation/getting-paid/Coding-at-the-AAP/Pages/Vaccine-Coding.aspx

American Academy of Family Physicians Vaccine Champion Report
- American Academy of Family Physicians Child and Adolescent Immunization Office Champions Project: www.aafp.org/content/dam/AAFP/documents/patient_care/immunizations/office-champions-final-report.pdf

One final caveat: insurance companies are starting to set limits on this kind of pediatric coding. For example, one company is only allowing 3 90461 codes per day, no matter how many vaccines the staff administers. This limitation can be frustrating because they are ignoring the intent of the CPT codes. However, it might require efforts at the level of the state legislature or medical academy to have an impact on these decisions.

SUMMARY

Providing vaccines places a significant logistical and financial burden on an office but is important in providing care to patients. Start the process by finding a vaccine champion, choosing a primary and backup vaccine coordinator, and creating a team in the office to promote and administer vaccines. Follow best practices when storing and monitoring vaccines. Create office policies for ordering vaccines in a fiscally sound manner, accepting deliveries, and managing inventory. Have backup processes in place to avoid preventable errors when administering vaccines. In addition, bill vaccine administration codes appropriately to collect the full reimbursement that is due. **Box 1** provides a list of key resources.

DISCLOSURE

The author has nothing to disclose.

REFERENCES

1. Ferdinands JM, Alyanak E, Reed C, et al. Waning of influenza vaccine protection: exploring the trade-offs of changes in vaccination timing among older adults. Clin Infect Dis 2019;70(8):1550–9.
2. CDC, Advisory Committee on Immunization Practices. Use of standing orders programs to increase adult vaccination rates. MMWR Recomm Rep 2000;49(RR01): 15–26.
3. CDC. Vaccination coverage among children aged 19-35 months - United States, 2017. MMWR Morb Mortal Wkly Rep 2018;67(40):1123–8.
4. Loehr J. Immunizations: how to protect patients and the bottom line. Fam Pract Manag 2015;22(2):24–9. Available at: https://www.aafp.org/fpm/2015/0300/p24.html. Accessed June 23, 2020.
5. CDC. General Best Practice Guidelines for Immunization: Available at: www.cdc.gov/vaccines/hcp/acip-recs/general-recs/downloads/general-recs.pdf. p. 71, 72. Accessed June 23, 2020.

Communicating About Immunizations

Jamie Loehr, MD

KEYWORDS

• Vaccine hesitancy • Communication about vaccines • Vaccine exemptions

KEY POINTS

- Vaccine hesitancy, defined as the desire to delay or defer immunizations, is present in a significant minority of patients and families.
- Vaccine hesitancy exists along a continuum, from patients with concerns and questions but who ultimately accept the recommended schedule to those who want to delay vaccines to those who refuse all vaccines.
- A strong recommendation and persistence are two strategies that have been shown to improve vaccination rates.
- Studies have shown that some communication strategies are not effective in increasing vaccination rates and might even be counterproductive.
- Removing personal and religious exemptions from vaccines required for school attendance has been shown to increase vaccination rates.

CONTENT

A majority of parents and patients are aware of, and accepting of, vaccinations. For encounters with them, a provider simply needs to state that a vaccine is due, review the benefits and possible side effects, and the patient or parent accepts the recommendation.

Vaccine hesitancy, however, is not uncommon in clinical practice, ranging from 8% of expectant mothers in Houston to 28% of respondents in the 2003 to 2004 National Immunization Survey.[1,2] Although it may appear to be a recent phenomenon, concerns about immunizations have been around for hundreds of years. Even Benjamin Franklin had questions about vaccinating his son against smallpox. He wrote in his autobiography:

> *In 1736 I lost one of my sons, a fine boy of four years old, by the smallpox taken in the common way. I long regretted bitterly and still regret that I had not given it to him by inoculation. This I mention for the sake of the parents who omit that operation, on the supposition that they should never forgive themselves if a child died*

Cayuga Family Medicine, 302 West Seneca Street, Ithaca, NY 14850, USA
E-mail address: Dr.Jamie.Loehr@Gmail.com

Prim Care Clin Office Pract 47 (2020) 419–430
https://doi.org/10.1016/j.pop.2020.05.010

under it; my example showing that the regret may be the same either way, and that, therefore, the safer should be chosen.[3]

DEFINING VACCINE HESITANCY

Vaccine hesitancy can be defined as the desire to defer or delay recommended immunizations despite easy access to the vaccines. This does not include situations where families want vaccines but cannot afford them and those where vaccines are unavailable. Fortunately, those situations are rare in the United States.

The most important thing to realize is that vaccine hesitancy exists along a spectrum. Some patients or parents are concerned but are reassured with additional information. Some accept the rationale behind vaccines but prefer a delayed schedule and ask to spread the immunizations out over time. A few patients or parents flatly refuse the vaccines, and some actively try to convert providers, telling them why they are wrong and why they should not be recommending vaccines at all.

To give some perspective, the vast majority of families accept the recommended vaccine schedule. In a telephone survey of 1500 parents of children aged 6 months to 23 months conducted in 2010, approximately 3% of the parents refused all vaccines. Approximately 20% of those parents, however, who accepted any vaccine delayed at least one vaccine.[4] That 20% of parents is the target audience for vaccine persuasion.

VACCINE HESITANCY IN THE TWENTY-FIRST CENTURY

The current wave of vaccine hesitancy started to spike in approximately the year 2000, due to a 1998 article, published in *The Lancet* by Dr Andrew Wakefield and colleagues, that linked the measles, mumps, and rubella (MMR) vaccine and autism.[5] The study was small, with only 12 children in the case series, and later was retracted by the journal. Dr Wakefield ultimately was found to have significant conflicts of interest that were not disclosed at the time of the publication and was stripped of his medical license for unethical and fraudulent conduct.[6]

Unfortunately, this article was widely publicized, with the result that thousands of parents have declined to vaccinate their children. Subsequently, several countries saw their level of measles immunization fall below the 95% vaccination threshold needed for herd immunity. Predictably, there were a resurgence of measles cases and some deaths.

Despite the debunking of the Wakefield study, and despite many studies since then showing no link between the MMR vaccine and autism, many families continue to have concerns about immunizations, and measles outbreaks continue. In the first several months of 2019, the United States had more than 1200 cases, the highest level in more than 25 years.[7]

Although measles might be the most prominent of vaccine-preventable disease outbreaks, other outbreaks have also occurred. In 2010, more than 9000 cases of pertussis were recorded in California and 10 children died, infants too young to have been vaccinated. Other pertussis outbreaks and deaths have been reported, including significant outbreaks in Minnesota, Vermont, Washington, and Wisconsin.[8]

WHAT CAN A PHYSICIAN DO?

Given the significant minority of parents and patients who are hesitant about vaccines, and given the serious consequences of these beliefs, it is clearly important to try to improve vaccine uptake in the office. On the positive side, there are some studies that show how simple interventions can lead to an uptick in vaccine acceptance. Some of these studies focus on managing the flow of patients in the office and some focus on managing vaccine hesitancy when it is present.

Start with a Strong Recommendation

To start, a strong recommendation from a physician is consistently the most important reason a parent or patient accepts the vaccination. Simply walking into the room and recommending the vaccine in a clear and concise manner increases the chance that the patient receives the vaccine that day. When asked why they did not receive a certain vaccine, many patients reply that their doctor did not recommend it to them.

There are many resources available on how to make a strong recommendation. Both the Centers for Disease Control and Prevention (CDC)[9] and the American Academy of Family Physicians[10] have video series that offer tips on recommending vaccines to patients. In addition, the CDC has a mnemonic, SHARE, that can be used in the room with patients:

- Share the tailored reasons why the recommended vaccine is right for a patient, given age, health status, lifestyle, occupation, or other risk factors.
- Highlight positive experiences with vaccines (personal or in the practice), as appropriate, to reinforce the benefits and strengthen confidence in vaccination.
- Address patient questions and any concerns about the vaccine, including side effects, safety, and vaccine effectiveness in plain and understandable language.
- Remind patients that vaccines protect them and their loved ones from many common and serious diseases.
- Explain the potential costs of getting the disease, including serious health effects, time lost (such as missing work or family obligations), and financial costs.[11]

Use a Presumptive Approach

Along with the strong recommendation, using a presumptive approach is more effective than using a participatory approach when recommending vaccines. The presumptive approach ("I recommend that your child receive three vaccines today.") matter-of-factly assumes that receiving the vaccines is the default position. This approach was associated with less parental resistance and a higher vaccine acceptance rate.[12]

The participatory approach ("Which vaccines do you want your child to receive today?") opens up the option of not receiving some or all of the vaccines. Although the participatory approach may be valid in many areas of medicine, it is less useful here. The data behind immunizations are so conclusive and the recommendation is so strong that providers do not want to suggest that not receiving vaccines is a good idea. Instead, providers want to clearly state that vaccines are safe, effective, and the standard in society.

It is also important to remember that vaccine hesitancy is a spectrum and concerns and questions should not be equated with complete refusal to vaccinate. Often a provider can easily answer the questions and move onto providing the vaccine.

Persistence

If a parent or patient declines a vaccine, do not be afraid to bring it up again later. Persistence is appropriate in this situation; 33% to 47% of parents who initially refused vaccinations for their children finally agreed at a subsequent appointment.[13]

Do not be afraid to use all available resources. Vaccine recommendations should come from everyone in the office. The front desk staff can mention that flu vaccines are available when checking a patient in for an appointment. The medical assistant can remind parents of required vaccinations for school entry. Everyone should be involved.

Standing Orders

Standing orders have been shown to increase vaccine uptake. Standing orders allow vaccines be given to a patient based on a written protocol instead of an individual patient order. There have been some dramatic improvements in vaccination rates when standing orders have been used in nursing homes and hospitals. Pneumococcal vaccination rates have gone from 2% to 83% in 1 facility and influenza vaccination rates went from 17% to 40% in a different facility. Even in ambulatory care centers, immunization rates were approximately 20% higher with the standing order program compared to when patient-specific reminders were used.[14]

Start Recommendations Early

Another communication technique that has been shown to improve vaccine rates is starting early. In a cluster randomized controlled trial of pregnant women in Japan, the intervention group received stepwise, interactive education about infant immunizations prenatally, postnatally, and 1 month after birth. The control group received a leaflet with general information about immunization. At 6 months of age, the infants of the intervention group women had a higher rate of completed vaccinations compared with the control group.[15]

Motivational Interviewing

There are other recommended approaches to communicating with vaccine-hesitant patients and parents. One method is to use motivational interviewing. This has been shown to work in other areas of medicine, such as lifestyle changes and smoking cessation.

Motivational interviewing starts with empathy, showing that the provider understands where the patient or parent is coming from. It helps to seek common ground by using phrases, such as "We both want the best for your child."

The next steps include looking for discrepancies in their beliefs ("If your child gets hospitalized with measles that might not be in their best interest."), adjusting to resistance without directly confronting the patient, and supporting self-efficacy. In the end, the patient or parent makes a final decision.

Motivational interviewing is especially good at respecting patient choices and building up trust in the physician patient relationship. Many experts feel that a foundation of trust is critical to vaccine acceptance in vaccine-hesitant families.

MANAGING PARENTAL CONCERNS

Another common approach to communicating about vaccine hesitancy is to discuss the concerns of the parents directly. There are several common concerns or beliefs that parents and patients express that lead to delayed vaccination. These include

1. Fear of side effects, such as autism or autoimmune disease
2. Fear of ingredients, such as thimerosal or aluminum
3. A perception that vaccine-preventable diseases are not serious
4. Mistrust of governments and/or pharmaceutical companies
5. Concerns about overloading the immune system with too many vaccines
6. Preference for the risks of natural disease over those of manufactured vaccinations

Using Data to Address Specific Concerns

Some experts feel that addressing fear-based beliefs with data and studies is the best approach. With this in mind, the provider can address the fear of side effects by emphasizing that long-term studies have found no increased significant side effects from any vaccine.

For example, with respect to autism and the MMR vaccine, the original Wakefield study included only 12 patients. Multiple large studies involving thousands of patients in the past 10 to 15 years have shown no association of autism with the MMR vaccine. This is the natural process of the scientific method, where small original studies might have positive findings that are not borne out by subsequent larger and more rigorous studies.

Discussing Aluminum

Along the same lines, the clinician could discuss the data behind aluminum in vaccines. First of all, infants receive more aluminum in their diet than they do in vaccines. Secondly, there is a reason for aluminum in vaccine: it provokes a better immune response. Finally, there are two medical conditions where excess aluminum can lead to consequences: significant renal disease or use of prolonged total parenteral nutrition in neonates. Otherwise, excess aluminum is excreted from the body via the urine or stool.

Using Big Data

Parents often use anecdotal evidence to link a side effect to a vaccine. This is difficult to refute in the specific circumstance. One way to approach this dilemma is to point out that certain health problems can happen randomly. The key question is whether they happen more commonly after a child is given a vaccine compared with children who have not received that vaccine.

Large studies are helpful. There are databases of tens of thousands of patients that are able to compare whether there are more fevers, syncope, or seizures after receiving a certain vaccine than in patients who did not receive that vaccine. Some individual studies exceed 30,000 patients. With few exceptions, there are no significant side effects after receiving vaccines. And for those few exceptions, they are well documented and clearly discussed in the vaccine information sheets that are available for each vaccine.

Addressing Side Effects

Any discussion should not obscure the fact that there are real side effects of vaccines. Some of them are significant. Approximately 1 in 25,000 to 1 in 40,000 children who receive the MMR vaccine develops idiopathic thrombocytopenic purpura, a temporary problem with low platelets, and some of these children are hospitalized.[16,17]

Most side effects of vaccines, however, are mild and short-lived. These include fevers, myalgias, and pain in the injected extremity. Acknowledging the real side effects but emphasizing the mild and transient character of most side effects, and putting the side effects in context with the benefits of the vaccine might help persuade some vaccine-hesitant families or patients.

COGNITIVE BIASES

Other experts feel that sharing data with vaccine-hesitant patients is beside the point. They point out that human psychology and cognitive biases are more important than data in the vaccine-hesitant mind. One common cognitive bias is the confirmation bias, a tendency to accept facts that fit prior beliefs and to discount facts that go

Table 1
Cognitive biases

Bias	Definition	Ways to Address in the Office
Confirmation bias	Accepting new information only if confirming existing beliefs and ignoring information that challenges those beliefs	Tailor vaccine recommendations to match current belief system (if possible). "I understand that you value purity and cleanliness. This vaccine will avoid a disease that will harm the body."
Status quo bias	Preferring choices that maintain the current state; avoiding change	Define the "current state" using a national perspective. "A vast majority of parents in the United States vaccinate their children using the CDC schedule."
Loss aversion bias	Losses have a larger psychological impact than gains. Thus, the risks of a vaccine have an outsized emotional response compared with the benefits.	Focus on the risks of the disease being prevented by the vaccine. "I know you have a lot planned this winter and don't have time to get sick. Avoiding the flu by getting the shot today could keep you well so you don't miss any days off work."
Availability bias	Placing greater importance on easily accessible or recently viewed information	Provide recent information in favor of vaccines in the waiting room, such as deaths from MMR in Samoa in December 2019.
Anchoring bias	Placing greater importance on the first piece of information received for a given topic	Provide information in favor of vaccines far in advance of the time the vaccine is needed. For example, discuss infant vaccines during pregnancy and human papillomavirus vaccine before age 11–12 y.

against those beliefs. Other important cognitive biases that play a role in the vaccine debate are included in **Table 1**.

There also are some biases that relate to how risks are perceived. One is the compression bias and another is the availability bias. The compression bias causes people to overestimate the frequency of rare risks. Specifically, risks of approximately 1 in 1000 are considered similar to risks on the order of 1,000,000 and are lumped together as pretty rare. There is a 1000-fold difference, however, between those two risks, which is significant on a population basis.

The availability bias leads to an overestimation of the frequency of rare events. If something unusual is reported in the media after someone receives a vaccine, it might seem much more common than it actually is. Taken in combination, the compression bias and the accessibility bias might lead to a sense that rare side effects are more common than the studies show.

UNDERSTANDING VALUES

Finally, other experts emphasize the values and the belief system of the patient or parent who is vaccine hesitant. There is some evidence that people who care more about purity and cleanliness are more vaccine hesitant because they do not want to put impure ingredients into their body. A way to approach this belief system might be to emphasize that the disease is unclean and the vaccine prevents that consequence.

CONSEQUENCES OF THE DISEASE ITSELF

Returning to the common concerns about vaccines, many vaccine-hesitant patients and parents feel that the vaccine-preventable diseases are not severe. However, some of these diseases can be deadly. In 2019, during the measles epidemics in the United States, some physicians felt that measles was a normal childhood disease with few if any serious consequences. Even in developed countries, however, approximately 20% of all patients infected with measles are hospitalized. More concerning, approximately 1 in 1000 patients can die from this infection and sometimes rate this can be much higher. In December 2019, Samoa faced an epidemic with more than 1400 cases (in a population of 200,000) and 70 deaths, with a majority of the deaths occurring in children under age 5 years. This is a fatality rate of approximately 5%.

Another example of the severity of disease is the *Haemophilus influenzae* bacteria (HIB). In the early 1980s, this bacterium caused approximately 20,000 cases of invasive disease in the United States and led to devastating consequences, including deafness, permanent neurologic disability, and death. In 1987, the HIB vaccine was introduced in the United States. By 1995, the incidence of invasive disease dropped by more than 99% to fewer than 100 cases a year. This vaccine wiped out a major disease of children.

More importantly, in countries where HIB vaccine is not routine, HIB is a major cause of lower respiratory infections. This goes to the theory that the disease is not important because it is not around. The bacterium is not common in the United States, however, because children are vaccinated against HIB as infants. Without the vaccine, invasive HIB disease would return to the United States.

OVERLOADING THE IMMUNE SYSTEM

Another common concern expressed by vaccine-hesitant parents is that too many vaccines overload the immune system. The current vaccine schedule protects against 8 diseases in the first 6 months of life. Including booster doses, infants might receive 25 doses of vaccines during that time period. The actual antigenic load, however, is less than in the past. The cellular pertussis vaccine of the 1990s had more than 3000 antigens but the current acellular pertussis vaccine has fewer than 5. The current load of those 25 doses is less than 300 antigens.

More importantly, immunocompetent infants theoretically are able to manage more than one million antigenic exposures. It is clear that the immune system can handle the extra burden from vaccines. In fact, there is some evidence that a higher antigenic load is linked to better performance on tests for attention and executive function at ages 7 years to 10 years. It might be true that more vaccines lead to fewer developmental delays.[18]

WHOM DO YOU TRUST?

Vaccine-hesitant patients and parents also are concerned about the influence of the vaccine manufacturers and governments in the vaccine recommendation process. Common concerns are that the pharmaceutical companies care only about profits and that the governmental agencies are beholden to the manufacturers.

The Centers for Disease Control and Prevention

Although a healthy skepticism of the process is appropriate, a few counter-examples might give some reassurance. In 1998, a rotavirus vaccine called RotaShield came on the market. Within a few months, the vaccine surveillance process noted an increase in the number of intussusceptions. The incidence was still rare, approximately 1 in 10,000 doses of vaccine, but it was higher than the baseline rate of 1 in 100,000 children per year. When this evidence came to light, the CDC committee on vaccines (Advisory Committee on Immunization Practices [ACIP]) recommended that the vaccine be removed from the market.

Another example happened in 2015. For several years, approximately 2004 to 2008, the live attenuated influenza vaccine outperformed the inactivated influenza vaccine in children under 8 years old. For several years after 2008, however, the live attenuated influenza vaccine performed poorly again some strains of the virus. Given these data, the ACIP recommended the live attenuated influenza vaccine not be used. Once again, the ACIP acted on the data to make recommendations.

The Food and Drug Administration

The Food and Drug Administration also has a role to play in vaccine recommendations. It is charged with ensuring that the vaccines are safe and effective. It places significant restrictions on the vaccine manufacturing process. For example, if a manufacturer wants to change the rubber stopper at the top of the vial of vaccine, it needs to wait three years to prove that the vaccine potency is not affected by the change. Vaccine manufacturing is one of the most regulated industries in the United States.

BUT DO THESE RECOMMENDED COMMUNICATIONS WORK?

One problem with all these suggestions on how to communicate with vaccine-hesitant patients, however, is that there is little evidence behind the recommendations. It often is true in medicine that what seems to be common sense might not hold up in critical studies. So although it might be believed that giving data to parents about vaccine manufacturing, side effects, or safety profiles is a useful process, it is not clear that it actually makes a difference.

For example, in a review of published reviews on strategies to address vaccine hesitancy, the summary statement includes the following: "From the literature, there is no strong evidence to recommend any specific intervention to address vaccine hesitancy/refusal."[19] And a randomized trial of physician communicating training at 56 clinics and involving 347 mothers came to the conclusion that "this physician target communication intervention did not reduce maternal hesitancy or improve physician self-efficacy. Research is needed to identify physician communication strategies effective at reducing parental vaccine hesitancy in the primary care setting"[20]

IS COMMUNICATION ACTUALLY COUNTERPRODUCTIVE?

More importantly, there is some concern that some communication techniques can backfire. In a 2014 study published in *Pediatrics*, more than 1700 parents were randomly assigned to 1 of 4 interventions or a control group. The interventions included the following: "(1) information explaining the lack of evidence that MMR causes autism from the Centers for Disease Control and Prevention; (2) textual information about the dangers of the diseases prevented by MMR from the Vaccine Information Statement; (3) images of children who have diseases prevented by the MMR vaccine; (4) a dramatic narrative about an infant who almost died of measles from a Centers for Disease Control and Prevention fact sheet."

The results were stunning. None of the interventions increased the intent to vaccinate and some actually decreased the intent to vaccinate. The group shown images of children with a vaccine-preventable disease had an increased belief of the connection between vaccines and autism. The group exposed to the dramatic narrative has a higher level of concerns about serious vaccine side effects.

The conclusions speak for themselves: "Current public health communications about vaccines may not be effective. For some parents, they actually may increase misperceptions or reduce vaccination intention. Attempts to increase concerns about communicable diseases or correct false claims about vaccines may be especially likely to be counterproductive. More study of pro-vaccine messaging is needed."[21]

REMOVING VACCINE EXEMPTIONS

There is another proven way to increase vaccination rates: removing vaccine exemptions. All states have regulations that students need to receive certain vaccines in order to attend public school. Some states have similar requirements regarding day care attendance as well.

In addition, all states allow medical exemptions to those school requirements. If a child is allergic to a component in a vaccine or if the child has a medical condition, such as immunosuppression from chemotherapy, that makes the vaccine unsafe, that child is exempt from receiving that vaccine but still can attend school.

However, many states allow religious exemptions to vaccines and a minority of states allow parents to express personal or philosophic exemptions to vaccines. There are several problems with these exemptions.

Problems with Exemptions

First of all, there is clear evidence that the more exemptions that are allowed in a given area the more likely there will be an outbreak of disease. In one study in Michigan, there was a clear link between clusters of nonmedical exemptions in given census tracts and the incidence of pertussis in those communities.[22] In Colorado, counties with more personal exemptions to vaccines also had more cases of measles and pertussis.[23]

The issue of clustering is especially important. On a statewide basis, the level of total exemptions usually is approximately 2% to 3% and in some states as high as 7%.[24] Certain geographic pockets, however, can have higher exemption rates. Drilling down to individual schools, some schools have more than 40% of their students lacking any immunizations. This geographic pattern is especially risky for disease outbreaks.

Secondly, most major religions support vaccinations.[25] In the United States, only Christian Science and the Dutch Reformed Church actively discourage immunizations and, in both communities, individuals are free to make their own decisions and vaccinate if they so choose. Internationally, some Islamic communities oppose vaccinations due to the presence of pork byproducts but, in the United States, the consensus of the Islamic community is that the benefits of vaccines make them acceptable under Islamic law.

Effect of Removing Exemptions

As of publication, there are five states that allow only medical exemptions: California, Maine, Mississippi, New York, and West Virginia. The lesson in California is most instructive. After they removed religious and personal exemptions in 2015, "the rate of kindergartners without up-to-date vaccination status decreased from 9.84% during 2013…to 4.87% during 2017."[26]

New York State removed the religious exemption in 2019. Before then, most parents with religious exemptions held strong personal beliefs that they felt were at the level of a religious belief. When the state removed the religious exemption, however, it was observed that most of those families agreed to vaccinate their children in order to have them remain in school.

Care needs to be taken, however, about unintended consequences of removing vaccine exemptions. Some families have decided to homeschool their children instead of accepting the immunization requirements. This may lead to more clustering of unimmunized children and actually may increase the risk of disease outbreaks. It can only be hoped that the increased numbers of children vaccinated outweigh the theoretical increased risk from clustering.

SUMMARY

In summary, remember

- A vast majority of patients and parents vaccinate themselves and their children.
- Vaccine hesitancy is a spectrum, and concerns and questions should not be equated with complete refusal to vaccinate.
- A vast majority of vaccine-hesitant families end up vaccinating their children.
- A strong recommendation from a physician is the most important reason that patients and parents vaccinate.
- Standing orders have been shown to increase vaccination rates.
- Unfortunately, most communication techniques aimed at increasing vaccination rates have not been shown to be effective and actually may be counterproductive.
- In the end, it may turn out that the most effective communication with regard to improving immunization uptake would be to work state legislatures to encourage the removal of all nonmedical exemptions.

DISCLOSURE

The author has nothing to disclose.

REFERENCES

1. Cunningham RM, Minard CG, Guffey D, et al. Prevalence of vaccine hesitancy among expectant mothers in Houston, Texas. Acad Pediatr 2018;18(2):154–60.
2. Gust DA, Darling N, Kennedy A, et al. Parents with doubts about vaccines: which vaccines and reasons why. Pediatrics 2008;122(4):718–25.
3. Best M, Katamba A, Neuhauser D. Making the right decision: Benjamin Franklin's son dies of smallpox in 1736. Qual Saf Health Care 2007;16(6):478–80.
4. McCauley MM, Kennedy A, Basket M, et al. Exploring the choice to refuse or delay vaccines: a national of parents of 6-through 23-month-olds. Acad Pediatr 2012;12(5):375–83.
5. Wakefield AJ, Murch SH, Anthony A, et al. RETRACTED: Ileal-lymphoid-nodular hyperplasia, non-specific colitis, and pervasive developmental disorder in children. Lancet 1998;351:637–41.
6. Rao TS, Andrade C. The MMR vaccine and autism: sensation, refutation, retraction, and fraud. Indian J Psychiatry 2011;53(2):95–6.

7. Patel M, Lee AD, Clemmons NS, et al. National update on measles cases and outbreaks — United States, January 1–October 1, 2019. MMWR Morb Mortal Wkly Rep 2019;68:893–6.
8. Based on information in CDC. Notice to readers: final 2012 Reports of Nationally Notifiable Infectious Disease. MMWR Morb Mortal Wkly Rep 2013;62(33):669–82. CDC, National Center for Immunization and Respiratory Diseases, Division of Bacterial Disease. 2012 Final Pertussis Surveillance Report. Available at: https://www.cdc.gov/pertussis/downloads/pertuss-surv-report-2012.pdf. Accessed September 29, 2019.
9. CDC, #HowIRecommend vaccination video series. Available at: https://www.cdc.gov/vaccines/howirecommend/index.html. Accessed December 15, 2019.
10. AAFP, conversations: improving adult immunizations rates using simple and strong recommendations. Available at: https://www.aafp.org/patient-care/public-health/immunizations/video.html. Accessed December 15, 2019.
11. CDC, standards for practice: vaccine recommendation. Available at: https://www.cdc.gov/vaccines/hcp/adults/for-practice/standards/recommend.html. Accessed December 15, 2019.
12. Opel DJ, Heritage J, Taylor JA, et al. The architecture of provider-parent vaccine discussions at health supervision visits. Pediatrics 2013;132(6):1037–46.
13. Edwards KM, Hackell JM, The Committee on Infectious Diseases, The Committee on Practice and Ambulatory Medicine. Countering vaccine hesitancy. Pediatrics 2016;138(3):e20162146.
14. McKibben LJ, Stange PV, Sneller VP, et al, Advisory Committee on Immunization Practices. Use of standing orders programs to increase adult vaccination rates. MMWR Recomm Rep 2000;49(RR-1):15–26.
15. Saitoh A, Saitoh A, Sato I, et al. Improved parental attitudes and beliefs through stepwise perinatal vaccination education. Hum Vaccin Immunother 2017;13(11):2639–45.
16. Black C, Kaye JA, Jick H. MMR vaccine and idiopathic thrombocytopaenic purpura. Br J Clin Pharmacol 2003;55(1):107–11.
17. CDC. Measles, Mumps, and Rubella (MMR) Vaccine Safety. Available at: https://www.cdc.gov/vaccinesafety/vaccines/mmr-vaccine.html. Accessed September 29, 2019.
18. Iqbal S, Barile JP, Thompson WW, et al. Number of antigens in early childhood vaccines and neuropsychological outcomes at age 7–10 years. Pharmacoepidemiol Drug Saf 2013;22:1263–70.
19. Dubé E, Gagnon D, MacDonald NE, et al. Strategies intended to address vaccine hesitancy: review of published reviews. Vaccine 2015;33(34):4191–203.
20. Henrikson NB, Opel DJ, Grothaus L, et al. Physician communication training and parental vaccine hesitancy: a randomized trial. Pediatrics 2015;136(1):70–9.
21. Nyhan B, Reifler J, Richey S, et al. Effective messages in vaccine promotion: a randomized trial. Pediatrics 2014;133(4):e835–42.
22. Omer SB, Enger KS, Moulton LH, et al. Geographic clustering of nonmedical exemptions to school immunization requirements and associations with geographic clustering of pertussis. Am J Epidemiol 2008;168(12):1389–96.
23. Feikin DR, Lezotte DC, Hamman RF, et al. Individual and community risks of measles and pertussis associated with personal exemptions to immunization. JAMA 2000;284(24):3145–50.
24. Mellerson J, Maxwell C, Knighton C, et al. Vaccination coverage for selected vaccines and exemption rates among children in Kindergarten - United States, 2017-18 School Year. MMWR Morb Mortal Wkly Rep 2018;67(40):1115–22.

25. Vanderbilt University Medical Center, Faculty & Staff Health and Wellness, Occupational Health Clinic. Immunizations and religion. 2013. Available at: https://www.vumc.org/health-wellness/news-resource-articles/immunizations-and-religion. Accessed September 29,2019.
26. Pingali SC, Delamater PL, Buttenheim AM, et al. Associations of statewide legislative and administrative interventions with vaccination status among Kindergartners in California. JAMA 2019;322(1):49–56.

Vaccine Safety

Laura Morris, MD, MSPH*, Sarah Swofford, MD, MSPH

KEYWORDS

• Vaccine safety • Vaccine adverse event • Vaccine event reporting • Vaccine injury • Vaccine injury compensation • Vaccine components

KEY POINTS

- Vaccines licensed for use in the United States undergo a rigorous safety program during development, manufacturing, distribution, and administration.
- Lay public concerns about vaccine components, such as aluminum, formaldehyde, and mercury, are not supported by research.
- The Vaccine Adverse Event Reporting System is part of a nationwide system to monitor for postmarketing adverse events from vaccines.
- The Vaccine Safety Datalink routinely monitors for adverse events from 8 participating health care organizations.
- The National Vaccine Injury Compensation Program provides funds to children injured by vaccines on a "no-fault" basis.

FIRST, DO NO HARM

Vaccine safety is a hot topic among patients, health care providers, and vaccine manufacturers and distributors. The success of modern immunization programs is evident: the incidence of many vaccine-preventable childhood illnesses has declined by more than 90%.[1] Along with this impressive reduction in morbidity and mortality comes a lack of public experience with the life-threatening sequelae of vaccine-preventable diseases and increased public scrutiny on vaccines' potential side effects and adverse reactions. Unlike medications prescribed to sick patients intended to make them well, vaccines are given to asymptomatic patients for primary prevention and thus must meet the highest possible standards to "first, do no harm" and, in fact, improve the health of the population as a whole.

VACCINE DEVELOPMENT: SAFETY FIRST

Vaccines licensed for use in the United States undergo a rigorous safety program during development, manufacturing, distribution, and administration; this includes

Department of Family & Community Medicine, University of Missouri, MA303 School of Medicine, One Hospital Drive, Columbia, MO 65212, USA
* Corresponding author.
E-mail address: morris6703@gmail.com

Prim Care Clin Office Pract 47 (2020) 431–441
https://doi.org/10.1016/j.pop.2020.04.001 primarycare.theclinics.com

careful regulatory oversight of clinical trials and several nationwide monitoring systems designed to capture postdistribution safety signals.[2]

In the United States, the Center for Biologics Evaluation and Research of the Food and Drug Administration (FDA) licenses all medications, including vaccines. Before licensing, manufacturers perform meticulous safety testing of all vaccine components. Manufacturers report safety data regarding adverse events alongside vaccine effectiveness for consideration during the process of vaccine licensure.[3]

Vaccines under development typically begin by testing in a basic science laboratory and proceed to animal testing after in vitro parameters are met. Once animal testing appears successful, vaccines progress through the 4 stages of clinical trials, similar to testing for a new medication for treatment of disease. Developers must submit plans for the trial and receive approval from safety and ethics review boards before beginning any research.[4]

The first 3 phases occur before vaccine licensure, and phase IV clinical trials occur after marketing. Observational research studies include long-term follow-up data after vaccines are licensed and administered to patients. Phase I trials are conducted with a few dozen adult volunteers and focus on identifying any possible side effects of the medication as well as any dose response. Vaccines intended to protect children are first tested in adults to identify any potential serious side effects before moving to include children in later phases of testing. Phase II trials include a few hundred patients and identify the appropriate dose of a vaccine needed to elicit an immune response. More safety data are also collected in phase II related to the frequency of side effects. In phase III trials, new vaccines are compared with placebo or another vaccine to identify additional side effects. Thousands of patients participate in phase III trials.

Only if the benefits of a vaccine substantially outweigh any potential risk for side effects does the FDA license the vaccine for use in the public. No medication, including vaccines, is guaranteed to be 100% effective and completely free from potential adverse effects. Rare side effects, such as those occurring in 1 out of hundreds of thousands of patients, may not appear until after wider distribution of the vaccine[4] (**Table 1**).

The FDA inspects vaccine manufacturing sites frequently to ensure the safety of the vaccine supply. Vaccines are produced in large lots, which are also tested to safeguard against contamination or loss of potency.[5,6]

FROM LICENSURE TO RECOMMENDATIONS

After licensure by the FDA, a vaccine is reviewed by the Advisory Committee on Immunization Practices (ACIP), a group of scientists and medical professionals tasked by the Centers for Disease Control and Prevention (CDC) to review research and make recommendations about public health and vaccine safety. The ACIP members represent major medical societies as well as government public health agencies. The ACIP does *not* include representatives from any pharmaceutical companies.[7] The ACIP-recommended vaccine schedule is reviewed and approved by the Director of the CDC and the Department of Health and Human Services and then published. The ACIP vaccine schedule is widely followed by US health care systems, practicing physicians, and other vaccine providers.[8]

POSTLICENSURE MONITORING OF VACCINE SAFETY

Before licensure, vaccines are used in thousands of people who are generally healthy. After vaccines are licensed, they are used in millions of people, some of whom are not healthy, and not always at the ideal time, so more rare adverse events may be

Table 1
Stages of clinical research for vaccine development

	Duration of Trials	Number/Type of Patients	Investigation Goals/Trial Outcomes
Phase I	<1 y	<100 adults	Dose response, major safety concerns
Phase II	1–2 y	100–300 adults	Dose response, efficacy/immunogenicity
Phase III	1–5 y	1000–3000 adults and children	Long-term efficacy/immunogenicity, coadministration with other vaccines, safety concerns
Phase IV	>1 y	>1000 postmarketing, adults and children	Long-term effectiveness, uncommon side effects, subtle safety signals
Observational studies	Long term	Millions of vaccine recipients	Long-term effectiveness, rare side effects

detected. In order to assess the safety of the vaccine, postlicensure surveillance is needed and is conducted through a variety of programs.

NATIONAL CHILDHOOD VACCINE INJURY ACT

Congress passed the National Childhood Vaccine Injury Act (NCVIA) in 1986 in response to increasing litigation surrounding vaccines and a resulting shortage of vaccine manufacturers willing to continue making vaccines.[9] During the mid-1970s, several patients filed lawsuits against vaccine manufacturers and providers alleging injuries from the diphtheria, tetanus, pertussis (DTP). Damages were awarded despite a lack of scientific evidence to support these claims, and as a result 2 of the last 3 manufacturers of DTP withdrew from the market, causing shortages of the DTP vaccine. Congress responded to the vaccine shortage and concerns from public health officials about outbreaks by passing the NCVIA, which established the National Vaccine Program Office to coordinate the CDC, FDA, National Institutes of Health, and Health Resources and Services Administration regarding immunizations.[5] It also requires health care providers to provide a vaccine information statement (VIS) to the person getting the vaccine or the guardian in the case of a child. A VIS must be given with every vaccination and contains a brief description of the disease as well as the risks and benefits of the vaccine.

The NCVIA also requires health care providers to report certain adverse events following vaccination to the Vaccine Adverse Event Reporting System (VAERS).

Under the NCVIA, the National Vaccine Injury Compensation Program (VICP) was created to compensate those injured by vaccines on a "no-fault" basis.

Info-box

National Childhood Vaccine Injury Act of 1986

- Established VAERS
- Required VIS with each vaccine
- Providers required to report certain adverse events to VAERS
- Created National VICP

VACCINE ADVERSE EVENT REPORTING SYSTEM

In the United States, the VAERS is a national early warning system to detect possible safety problems. It is comanaged by the CDC and the FDA.[5] VAERS receives reports from physicians, manufacturers, patients and their families, or anyone else who chooses to report a case. VAERS is a passive reporting system, meaning it relies on individuals to send in reports. Reports may be submitted by phone, fax, mail, or online (preferred) at https://vaers.hhs.gov/reportevent.html. VAERS is not designed to determine if a vaccine caused a health problem, but it is useful for detecting unusual or unexpected patterns of adverse event reporting that might indicate a possible safety problem with a vaccine.[10]

In addition, the NCVIA requires health care providers to report (1) any adverse event listed by the manufacturer as a contraindication to further doses of the vaccine; or (2) any adverse event listed in the VAERS table of reportable events following vaccination that occurs within the specified time period (**Table 2**).

The CDC and FDA use several methods to analyze VAERS data, looking for concerning patterns or unusual or unexpected changes in adverse event reporting that

Table 2
Excerpt from Vaccine Adverse Event Reporting System table of reportable events

VAERS Table of Reportable Events Following Vaccination*

Vaccine/Toxoid	Event and Interval** from Vaccination
Tetanus in any combination: DTaP, DTP, DTP-Hib, DT, Td, TT, Tdap, DTaP-IPV, DTaP-IPV/Hib, DTaP-HepB-IPV	A. Anaphylaxis or anaphylactic shock (7 d) B. Brachial neuritis (28 d) C. Shoulder injury related to vaccine administration (7 d) D. Vasovagal syncope (7 d) E. Any acute complications or sequelae (including death) of above events (interval, not applicable) F. Events described in manufacturer's package insert as contraindications to additional doses of vaccine (interval, see package insert)

* Effective date: March 21, 2017. The Reportable Events Table (RET) reflects what is reportable by law (42 USC 300aa-25) to the Vaccine Adverse Event Reporting System (VAERS) including conditions found in the manufacturer package insert. In addition, healthcare professionals are encouraged to report any clinically significant or unexpected events (even if not certain the vaccine caused the event) for any vaccine, whether or not it is listed on the RET. Manufacturers are also required by regulation (21CFR 600.80) to report to the VAERS program all adverse events made known to them for any vaccine.
** Represents the onset interval between vaccination and the adverse event.
From Vaccine Adverse Event Reporting System. Table of reportable events. Available at: https://vaers.hhs.gov/docs/VAERS_Table_of_Reportable_Events_Following_Vaccination.pdf.

might indicate a safety problem in a specific vaccine or vaccine type.[11] CDC and FDA physicians, epidemiologists, and statisticians review reports on the most common adverse events, current versus historical data, and reporting trends over time, such as comparing adverse events from influenza vaccines across multiple influenza seasons. They use vaccine doses distributed as a proxy measure for persons vaccinated and can approximate rates of adverse events in that context. However, because VAERS is a passive, numerator-only surveillance system, it is not able to provide incidence of adverse events. The proportion of reports involving a specific adverse event and a specific vaccine can be compared with the proportion of reports involving the same adverse event and other vaccines, and using disproportionality analyses can determine adverse events more frequently associated with a particular vaccine. CDC and FDA physicians also conduct clinical reviews of serious reports and selected reports based on descriptive analysis.

Strengths of the VAERS include the large and diverse population that is available to report (the entire US population), which makes the system able to rapidly detect possible safety problems and rare adverse events. VAERS can often provide early information on potential vaccine safety problems, because of the direct reporting capability and speed at which reports and follow-up information can be processed and analyzed, and is less impacted by data lags than claims-based monitoring systems. VAERS data are made available online to the public, providing transparency regarding vaccine safety. Weaknesses of the VAERS center on reporting bias, including underreporting of common and mild adverse events, and stimulated reporting, which is increased reporting in response to media attention or increased public awareness of a particular adverse event. Because VAERS data do not include an unvaccinated comparison group, it is not possible to calculate the risk of an adverse event in vaccinated versus unvaccinated individuals. Finally, it generally cannot be determined using VAERS data if the vaccine caused an adverse event (just that they are associated).

Exceptions would be unambiguous biologically plausible cases (pain and redness at the injection site) or when the vaccine strain of the virus was isolated from ill individuals and is known to be genetically distinct from the wild-type virus strain.[12]

VACCINE ADVERSE EVENT REPORTING SYSTEM IN ACTION

VAERS received 19,760 reports following the human papillomavirus (HPV) quadrivalent vaccine from 2006 to 2009.[13] Of these reports, 94% were nonserious (dizziness, syncope, and injection site reaction), and there were no new or unexpected safety concerns.

VAERS received 108 confirmed cases of intussusception following oral rotavirus vaccine from 2008 to 2014 with a clustering observed on days 3 to 8 after dose 1, with an excess risk estimated at 1.2 to 2.8 per 100,000.[14] This finding is in contrast to an annual decline of 40,000 gastroenteritis hospitalizations and an annual reduction of $140 million in treatment costs associated with rotavirus.

The recombinant zoster vaccine (RZV; Shingrix) was licensed by the FDA in October 2017. In prelicense clinical trials of 6773 participants, 85% reported local or systemic reactions, with ~17% experiencing grade 3 reactions (erythema or induration >10 cm in size or systemic symptoms that interfere with normal activity).[15] Rates of serious adverse events were similar in the RZV and placebo groups. During the first 8 months of use when 3.2 million doses were given, VAERS received a total of 4381 reports of adverse events, 3% of which were classified as serious. No unexpected patterns were detected in reports of adverse events or serious adverse events. Findings from the VAERS monitoring system were consistent with the safety profile in prelicensure trials.

VACCINE SAFETY DATALINK

The Vaccine Safety Datalink (VSD) is a collaboration between the CDC's Immunization Safety Office and 8 health care organizations (Kaiser Permanente Washington, Harvard Pilgrim Health Care Institute, HealthPartners Institute, Kaiser Permanente Northwest, Kaiser Permanente Northern California, Kaiser Permanente Colorado, Marshfield Clinic Research Institute, and Kaiser Permanente Southern California).[5] The VSD started in 1990 in order to monitor safety of vaccines and conduct studies about adverse events following immunization. The VSD uses electronic health data from each participating site, including the specific vaccine given to each patient, date of vaccination, other vaccines given on the same day, and diagnosis codes for medical encounters occurring in outpatient clinics, urgent care, emergency department, and hospital settings.[5] The VSD conducts vaccine safety studies based on questions or concerns raised from the medical literature or reports to the VAERS. The VSD monitors for possible adverse events when new vaccines are licensed or when there are changes in how a vaccine is given.

The VSD population represents 3% of the total US population or more than 9 million people annually.[16,17] A study comparing the 2010 VSD population with the 2010 US Census found the group to be representative of the general population, lending validity to the generalizability of VSD findings.[16] There were no major differences in sex, race, ethnicity, and educational level between the VSD group and the US population. There were slight differences in income estimates based on neighborhood (36% of VSD population earning less than $50,000 per year compared with 51% of US population), but the VSD had more than 2 million individuals in this lower-income group. The VSD population represents 1.1% of the US Medicaid population.

VSD researchers have also developed Rapid Cycle Analysis (RCA) as a complement to traditional retrospective studies. RCA consists of weekly monitoring to identify early signals of adverse events at a higher rate than expected. Further analysis of these signals determines if there is an increased risk of an adverse event following vaccination.[17] RCA has included seasonal influenza vaccines, rotavirus vaccine, and HPV vaccine. The RCA surveillance system detected a 2-fold increased risk of febrile seizures occurring 7 to 10 days after measles, mumps, rubella, and varicella (MMRV) vaccination in children 12 to 23 months old compared with separate measles, mumps, and rubella (MMR) and varicella vaccine.[18] The ACIP subsequently changed the recommendation from a preference for MMRV to no preference for either MMRV or separate MMR + varicella vaccines.

The RCA system was used for monitoring the safety of the 2009 pandemic H1N1 influenza vaccine. The initial VSD RCA findings, along with a review of VAERS reports that identified no safety signals, provided the public early reassuring data on the safety of this new vaccine.[17]

The VSD has been used to monitor the risk of adverse events from influenza vaccine across seasons.[19] VSD can also monitor outcomes that develop later in time, including a case-control study showing prenatal and early-life exposure to thimerosal-containing vaccines does not increase the risk of autism spectrum disorders.[20] VSD has the ability to study special populations, such as premature infants and pregnant women. VSD is effective in studying priority areas for vaccine safety, such as new vaccines, new recommendations related to existing vaccines, risk of specific clinical disorders associated with immunization (intussusception and rotavirus vaccine), and special populations (risk of spontaneous abortion in pregnant women after influenza vaccine, safety of tetanus, diphtheria, pertussis [Tdap] in the elderly).[17]

INSURANCE CLAIMS DATA

In addition to the previously described vaccine safety monitoring systems of the CDC and FDA, independent analysis of claims data from insurance companies provides additional data on safety of vaccines. Medicare claims data during the 2009 to 2010 influenza season showed no elevation in the rate of Guillain-Barre syndrome following seasonal or H1N1 influenza vaccination.[21] An observational cohort study using insurance claims from a commercially insured population of 57,000 infants receiving the rotavirus vaccine found no increased risk for intussusception, lower respiratory tract infection, Kawasaki disease, or mortality.[22]

NATIONAL VACCINE INJURY COMPENSATION PROGRAM

The national VICP was created in 1986 through the NCVIA passed by Congress, in response to lawsuits against vaccine manufacturers and health care providers that threatened to cause vaccine shortages and an increase in vaccine-preventable disease.[23] The purpose of the program is to ensure that individuals injured by certain vaccines are provided with fair and efficient compensation, and to support a stable vaccine supply by limiting liability for vaccine manufacturers and vaccine administrators. The VICP is a no-fault alternative to the traditional legal system for resolving vaccine injury claims. Any individual who received a covered vaccine (recommended by CDC for routine administration to children and pregnant women) and thinks they were injured as a result of the vaccine, can file a petition. Parents and guardians may file a petition on behalf of children. The US Department of Health and Human Services medical staff reviews the petition and determines if it meets medical criteria for compensation. The US Department of Justice then develops a report that includes the medical recommendation and legal analysis and submits it to the US Court of

Federal Claims. The Court then determines if the petitioner should be compensated, which is paid by the US Department of Health and Human Services.

According to the CDC, from 2006 to 2017, more than 3.4 billion doses of vaccines were distributed in the United States, with 6467 petitions to the VICP during this same time period, of which 4450 were compensated; this means for every 1 million doses of vaccine that were distributed, approximately 1 individual was compensated by the VICP.[24]

COMMON SAFETY CONCERNS OF THE PUBLIC

Because vaccines are typically given to healthy people, and most vaccines doses are administered to infants and children, a high level of scrutiny of vaccine formulations is important.

Aluminum

Many parents are concerned to see aluminum listed as a vaccine component. Aluminum is added to vaccines as an adjuvant to enhance the immune response to the active vaccine components, but the total amount of aluminum exposure remains very low.[25] Based on a 2011 study examining the childhood vaccine schedule, an infant may receive up to 4.2 mg of aluminum from vaccines during the first 12 months of life.[26] In comparison, a milk-based formula-fed infant will ingest up to 38 mg of aluminum, and a soy formula-fed infant will ingest up to 117 mg of aluminum.[27]

Thimerosal

Modern vaccines manufactured in the United States no longer contain thimerosal. Vaccine manufacturers removed this antimicrobial preservative agent from vaccines given to children less than 6 years of age at the request of several US health agencies, including the FDA and CDC.[28] Thimerosal contains low levels of ethylmercury, a naturally occurring mercurial compound, and does not contain toxic methylmercury (the form of the element that accumulates in fish). No studies have found evidence of a link between ethylmercury exposure and neurotoxicity or autism spectrum disorders.[29]

Formaldehyde

Another agent added to vaccines is formaldehyde. Formaldehyde, despite public perceptions, is also a naturally occurring substance present in the human body as well as in the indoor and outdoor environment.[30] Formaldehyde is used in vaccines to weaken toxins and deactivate live viruses. The amount of formaldehyde remaining in a vaccine at the end of the manufacturing process is negligible and is not a safety concern.[31]

PREVENTING VACCINE INJURY

In addition to national safety monitoring efforts, it is important for health care providers to take steps to prevent vaccine-related reactions or injuries for the individual patient.

Syncope is most commonly reported after routine adolescent vaccines, including HPV, MCV (meningococcal conjugate vaccine), and TdaP. The CDC has received reports of syncope after nearly all vaccines, but 63% of the VAERS reports during 2005 to 2007 were associated with these 3 routine adolescent vaccines.[32] Because the components of the vaccines are different, syncope is likely related to the procedure of receiving a vaccine rather than an adverse reaction to the vaccine component. Reported syncope occurred within 5 minutes of vaccination in 52%, and 70% of reported syncope occurred within 15 minutes. Syncope-related injuries can be serious, including head injuries from falls or motor vehicle accidents if syncope occurs while driving. All providers administering vaccinations to adolescents should be aware of the potential for syncope. ACIP recommends providers consider observing adolescents for 15 minutes after vaccination.

For patients with latex allergy, there are available lists of vaccine packaging that may contain latex. Immediate-type allergic reactions due to latex allergy have been described after vaccination, but are rare. If a patient has a severe anaphylactic allergy to latex, vaccines in vials or syringes that contain rubber latex should be avoided.[33] The CDC publishes a table of vaccine type and whether it contains latex (https://www.cdc.gov/vaccines/pubs/pinkbook/downloads/appendices/B/latex-table.pdf). If in doubt, check the manufacturer's package insert.

Providers commonly have questions from patients about egg allergy and safety of vaccines. Generally, a person who can eat eggs or egg products can receive vaccines that contain eggs, including the yellow fever and egg-containing influenza vaccines.[33] Studies have shown that children who have a history of severe allergy to eggs rarely have reactions to MMR vaccine, because the viruses are grown in chick embryo fibroblasts, not actually in eggs.[33] Current recommendations for influenza vaccine from the CDC indicate patients who have only experienced hives after exposure to eggs should receive any age-appropriate flu vaccine (IIV or LAIV4).[34] Patients who have a more serious reaction than hives to egg exposure (angioedema, respiratory distress, dizziness, require epinephrine, or emergency room visit) may also receive any flu vaccine, but the vaccine should be given in a medical setting and supervised by a health care provider who is able to manage severe allergic reactions.

DISCLOSURE

The authors have nothing to disclose.

REFERENCES

1. Roush SW, Murphy TV. Historical comparisons of morbidity and mortality for vaccine-preventable diseases in the United States. JAMA 2007;298(18):2155–63.
2. U.S. Food and Drug Administration. Vaccine safety & availability. 2019. Available at: https://www.fda.gov/vaccines-blood-biologics/safety-availability-biologics/vaccine-safety-availability. Accessed August 30,2019.
3. U.S. Food and Drug Administration. Ensuring the safety of vaccines in the United States. 2011. Available at: https://www.fda.gov/files/vaccines,%20blood%20&%20biologics/published/Ensuring-the-Safety-of-Vaccines-in-the-United-States.pdf. Accessed August 30,2019.
4. Centers for Disease Control and Prevention vaccines for your children. 2018. Available at: https://www.cdc.gov/vaccines/parents/index.html. Accessed September 20, 2019.
5. Centers for Disease Control and Prevention. Vaccine safety monitoring. 2016. Available at: https://www.cdc.gov/vaccinesafety/ensuringsafety/monitoring/index.html. Accessed August 30,2019.
6. World Health Organization. Principles and considerations for adding a vaccine to a national immunization programme. In: DeRoeck D, Wang SA, Department of Immunization, editors. From decision to implementation and monitoring. Geneva (Switzerland): World Health Organization; 2014. p. 99–103.
7. Centers for Disease Control and Prevention. Advisory committee on immunization practices policies and procedures 2018. Available at: https://www.cdc.gov/

vaccines/acip/committee/downloads/Policies-Procedures-508.pdf. Accessed September 20, 2019.
8. Pickering LK, Orenstein WA. Licensure, approval, and uptake of vaccines in the United States. J Pediatr Infect Dis Soc 2018;7(suppl_2). S46–s48.
9. Freed GL, Katz SL, Clark SJ. Safety of vaccinations. Miss America, the media, and public health. JAMA 1996;276(23):1869–72.
10. HHS contracts Sanofi pasteur for Zika vaccine development. Biopharm Int 2016; 29(10):52.
11. Shimabukuro TT, Nguyen M, Martin D, et al. Safety monitoring in the Vaccine Adverse Event Reporting System (VAERS). Vaccine 2015;33(36):4398–405.
12. Wharton M. Vaccine safety: current systems and recent findings. Curr Opin Pediatr 2010;22:88–93.
13. Arana JE, Harrington T, Cano M, et al. Post-licensure safety monitoring of quadrivalent human papillomavirus vaccine in the Vaccine Adverse Event Reporting System (VAERS), 2009–2015. Vaccine 2018;36(13):1781–8.
14. Haber P, Parashar UD, Haber M, et al. Intussusception after monovalent rotavirus vaccine-United States, Vaccine Adverse Event Reporting System VAERS, 2008-2014. Vaccine 2015;33(38):4873–7.
15. Hesse EM, Shimabukuro TT, Su JR, et al. Postlicensure safety surveillance of recombinant zoster vaccine (Shingrix)–United States, October 2017-June 2018. MMWR Morb Mortal Wkly Rep 2019;68(4):91–4.
16. Sukumaran L, McCarthy NL, Li R, et al. Demographic characteristics of members of the Vaccine Safety Datalink (VSD): a comparison with the United States population. Vaccine 2015;33(36):4446–50.
17. McNeil MM, Gee J, Weintraub ES, et al. The Vaccine Safety Datalink: successes and challenges monitoring vaccine safety. Vaccine 2014;32(42):5390–8.
18. Klein NP, Fireman B, Yih WK, et al. Measles-mumps-rubella-varicella combination vaccine and the risk of febrile seizures. Pediatrics 2010;126(1). e1–8.
19. Greene SK, Kulldorff M, Lewis EM, et al. Near real-time surveillance for influenza vaccine safety: proof-of-concept in the Vaccine Safety Datalink Project. Am J Epidemiol 2010;171(2):177–88.
20. Price CS, Thompson WW, Goodson B, et al. Prenatal and infant exposure to thimerosal from vaccines and immunoglobulins and risk of autism. Pediatrics 2010;126(4):656–64.
21. Burwen DR, Sandhu SK, MaCurdy TE, et al. Surveillance for Guillain-Barré syndrome after influenza vaccination among the medicare population, 2009-2010. Am J Public Health 2012;102(10):1921–7.
22. Hoffman V, Abu-Elyazeed R, Enger C, et al. Safety study of live, oral human rotavirus vaccine: a cohort study in United States health insurance plans. Hum Vaccin Immunother 2018;14(7):1782–90.
23. Health Resources & Services Administration. National Vaccine Injury Compensation Program. 2019. Available at: https://www.hrsa.gov/vaccine-compensation/index.html. Accessed September 19, 2019.
24. Health Resources & Services Administration. National Vaccine Injury Compensation Program: monthly statistics report. 2019. Available at: https://www.hrsa.gov/sites/default/files/hrsa/vaccine-compensation/data/data-statistics-september-2019.pdf. Accessed September 19, 2019.
25. Administration, U.S.F.a.D.. Common ingredients in U.S. licensed vaccines. 2019. Available at: https://www.fda.gov/vaccines-blood-biologics/safety-availability-biologics/common-ingredients-us-licensed-vaccines. Accessed September 20, 2019.

26. Mitkus RJ, King DB, Hess MA, et al. Updated aluminum pharmacokinetics following infant exposures through diet and vaccination. Vaccine 2011;29(51): 9538–43.
27. Vaccine ingredients–aluminum. Available at: https://www.chop.edu/centers-programs/vaccine-education-center/vaccine-ingredients/aluminum. Accessed September 20, 2019.
28. Thimerosal and vaccines. 2018. Available at: https://www.fda.gov/vaccines-blood-biologics/safety-availability-biologics/thimerosal-and-vaccines. Accessed September 20, 2019.
29. Hviid A, Stellfeld M, Wohlfahrt J, et al. Association between thimerosal-containing vaccine and autism. JAMA 2003;290:1763–6.
30. U.S. Food and Drug Administration. Common ingredients in U.S. licensed vaccines. 2018. Available at: https://www.fda.gov/vaccines-blood-biologics/safety-availability-biologics/common-ingredients-us-licensed-vaccines. Accessed September 20,2019.
31. What's in vaccines. 2019. Available at: https://www.cdc.gov/vaccines/vac-gen/additives.htm. Accessed September 20, 2019.
32. Centers for Disease Control and Prevention (CDC). Syncope after Vaccination-United States, 2005-2007. MMWR Morb Mortal Wkly Rep 57(17): 457-460.
33. Broder K, Vellozzi C, Weinbaum C, et al. Safety of influenza A (H1N1) 2009 monovalent vaccines—United States, October 1-November 24, 2009. MMWR Morb Mortal Wkly Rep 2009;58(48):1351–6.
34. Andrew MK, Bowles SK, Pawelec G, et al. Influenza vaccination in older adults: recent innovations and practical applications. Drugs Aging 2019;36(1):29–37.

Vaccinating in Pregnancy: Opportunities and Challenges

Alexandra Schieber, DO*, David O'Gurek, MD

KEYWORDS

• Immunization • Pregnancy • Preconception health

KEY POINTS

- Immunizations are a part of comprehensive preconception health to promote family-centered care and advance maternal-child health.
- Immunizations before and during pregnancy promote not only maternal health but also through passive immunity promote a healthy pregnancy and postnatal period.
- Certain immunizations are not indicated in pregnancy and therefore it is important to understand appropriate immunization care for patients who are pregnant.

GENERAL IMMUNOLOGY CONCEPTS IN PREGNANCY

A healthy immune system serves to shield the body from foreign organisms and their effects. Inherent in this system is the ability to distinguish self from nonself antigens. During pregnancy, the mother harbors an antigenically foreign fetus while still maintaining the ability to fight infection. A series of complex adaptations must occur within the maternal immune system to create a state of selective immune tolerance to the fetus for both the mother and the fetus to survive.[1]

One such adaptation is the presence of special maternal regulatory T cells that recognize fetal cells as foreign antigens and work to specifically suppress the maternal immune response to these cells. These are similar to the regulatory T cells that suppress the autoimmune response and prevent autoimmune disease. The specific nature of this response allows the maternal immune system to maintain its defenses and explains the phenomenon that certain autoimmune diseases seem to improve during pregnancy.[1] There are multiple other cell types involved, upregulation of certain immune functions and downregulation of others and alterations in immune cell quantity and phenotype during pregnancy to result ultimately in a remarkable balance allowing the fetus to grow unharmed while leaving maternal defenses intact.[2] As the

Department of Family & Community Medicine, Lewis Katz School of Medicine at Temple University, Jones Hall, 3rd Floor, 1316 West Ontario Street, Philadelphia, PA 19140, USA
* Corresponding author.
E-mail address: Alexandra.schieber@tuhs.temple.edu

Prim Care Clin Office Pract 47 (2020) 443–452
https://doi.org/10.1016/j.pop.2020.05.001

fetus develops, not only is it shielded from harm via these unique mechanisms, but it confers benefit and protection via maternal antibodies that are transmitted across the placenta mostly toward the end of pregnancy. Thus, despite a newborn infant's immature immune system, it is protected during the first months of life via maternal antibodies.

Maternal immunoglobulin (Ig)G is transported across the placenta starting at the beginning of the second trimester and continues to term, with most IgG transmission occurring during the third trimester, more specifically the last weeks of pregnancy. Very little IgG is transmitted during the first trimester. For maternal immunization to protect the newborn, adequate levels of IgG must be present in maternal circulation during this key period late in the pregnancy. The more IgG the fetus receives, the longer the immunity will last after birth.[3]

In the postpartum period, breastfeeding introduces further opportunity for the mother to transmit immunity to the neonate. Maternal IgA is transferred through breastmilk offering protection against enteric infection. This and other maternal antibodies appear to coat the infant's gut surface offering protection by enhancing the infant's immune response.[4]

Establishing good practice surrounding appropriately timed, safe vaccination before, during, and between pregnancies affords us opportunity to protect and strengthen the health of the maternal-fetal dyad throughout the continuum of preconception care, antenatal care, postpartum care, and care of the newborn infant. It also leaves tremendous space for growth in possibilities, including development of vaccines against Group B Streptococcus infection, respiratory syncytial virus, human immunodeficiency virus, and others.

IMMUNIZATION IN THE PRECONCEPTION PERIOD

Immunization and Preconception Health

Preconception health more broadly applies to the health of all individuals, regardless of gender identity, gender expression, or sexual orientation, during reproductive years.[5] Although the approach is often focused on healthy fertility and promoting maternal-child health, it more broadly applies to risk reduction, healthy lifestyle, and addressing readiness for pregnancy whether or not pregnancy is desired. Although a comprehensive approach to prevent preterm births, improve birth weight, prevent congenital anomalies, reduce infant mortality, and reduce maternal mortality,[6] preconception health includes assessment of vaccine-preventable illness risk factors as well as history of illness or vaccination to promote these same outcomes.[7] Although the focus often seems to center around maternal vaccination, it is critical to note that preconception immunization health includes partners as well, and therefore family-centered care is critical to ensuring preconception health.

Influenza Vaccination in the Preconception Period

Influenza vaccine is indicated for all individuals 6 months or older who do not have contraindications.[8] Vaccination for all individuals planning a pregnancy with inactivated influenza vaccine or live attenuated influenza vaccine during the influenza season is important given risks of complications of influenza during pregnancy,[9] as well as the added benefit of antibody transfer to the newborn.[10]

Tetanus, Diphtheria, and Acellular Pertussis Vaccination in the Preconception Period

Although assessing for up-to-date tetanus immunity is important for preconception health, vaccination with diphtheria-tetanus-pertussis vaccination is more important during pregnancy to provide the greatest benefit of passive immunity to the fetus. Although not directly linked with passive immunity, partner vaccination for both influenza and diphtheria-tetanus-pertussis are important. Preconception vaccination is important, as well as several vaccines that are not indicated during pregnancy, notably human papilloma virus (HPV) vaccine, varicella vaccine, and measles, mumps, and rubella (MMR) vaccine.

Immune Status Testing Before Pregnancy

The significance of hepatitis B during pregnancy is emphasized with universal screening of pregnant women for hepatitis B virus (HBV) with testing of hepatitis B surface antigen during the first trimester regardless of vaccination or testing previously. This is critical to identify precautions for delivery management as well as timely prophylaxis for infants born to mothers with hepatitis B.[11] Maternal varicella (chickenpox) has significant implications for pregnancy including congenital varicella syndrome (low birth weight and limb, ophthalmologic, and neurologic abnormalities) as well as neonatal varicella.[12] Therefore, screening for varicella immunity is recommended as part of routine preconception care. Mumps can affect male fertility and measles and rubella can affect a healthy pregnancy. Given that the MMR vaccine is a live vaccine, MMR should not be administered to individuals who are pregnant or who are hoping to soon become pregnant. Women should be counseled to avoid becoming pregnant for at least 28 days after receiving MMR (or other live attenuated vaccines) to avoid fetal risks.[13]

A review of vaccinations of importance for preconception health are outlined in **Table 1**.

IMMUNIZATION IN THE ANTENATAL PERIOD

Influenza and Adult Tetanus, Diphtheria, and Pertussis Vaccines

Understanding preconception health and the benefits of vaccination during this interval sheds light on immunization that occurs during the antenatal period. As noted, live vaccinations are contraindicated during pregnancy and therefore preconception care delivery provides an opportunity to ensure immunologic protection to promote a healthy pregnancy. Furthermore, inactivated influenza vaccination is recommended for individuals who will be pregnant during influenza season either before or during pregnancy. Diphtheria-tetanus-pertussis vaccination is indicated, specifically with adult tetanus, diphtheria, and pertussis (Tdap) administered from 27 through 36 weeks' gestation of each pregnancy given the benefits of passive immunity to the fetus conferring the highest potential IgG transmission during this time period.[14]

Additional Vaccination Considerations in the Antenatal Period

Although not universally provided, there are additional vaccinations that are recommended in specific populations during pregnancy. Meningococcal conjugate (MenACWY) and meningococcal serogroup B vaccination, although preferably administered before pregnancy, if indicated, pregnancy should not preclude vaccination. In addition, any individual at risk for hepatitis A or hepatitis B during pregnancy and wishes to be prevented may receive the vaccination[15,16]; however, this should also include discussion on additional methods to prevent both. HPV vaccination is not recommended during pregnancy; however, inadvertent vaccination has not been shown to have adverse outcomes.

Pneumococcal vaccination is recommended for adults with specific chronic health conditions with different indications for the 23-valent pneumococcal vaccine (PPSV23)

Table 1
Benefits of vaccinations as part of preconception care

Immunization	Preconception Health Benefits
Human papilloma virus (HPV) vaccine	• HPV infection associated with preterm birth and placental abnormalities.[27] • Procedures related to HPV and abnormal cervical cytology lead to cervical incompetence
Hepatitis B (HBV) vaccine	• Prevention of chronic HBV status with complications in patient • Reducing vertical transmission during pregnancy
Varicella vaccine	• Reducing risks of maternal varicella during pregnancy • Reducing risks to fetus including congenital varicella syndrome and neonatal varicella
Measles, mumps, rubella (MMR) vaccine	• Measles illness in pregnancy may be associated with increased rates of spontaneous abortion, premature labor and preterm delivery, and low birth weight[28] • Rubella infection during pregnancy, particularly during the first trimester can result is miscarriage, stillbirth, and CRS (cataracts, hearing loss, mental retardation, and congenital heart defects)[29]
Influenza vaccine	• Influenza during pregnancy associated with higher rates of complications, including increased risk of intensive care unit admission and adverse perinatal and neonatal outcomes[8]
Diphtheria-tetanus-pertussis vaccine	• Regardless of status, revaccination recommended during pregnancy for passive immunity

and the 13-valent pneumococcal vaccine (PCV13).[17] (**Table 2**)Although PPSV23 can be administered during pregnancy, there are currently no recommendations regarding administering PCV13 safely during pregnancy.

Due to their potential for significant fetal harm, if a nonimmune pregnant person is exposed to measles or varicella, postexposure prophylaxis may be given by administering Immune globulin within 6 days of exposure for measles and within 10 days of exposure for varicella.[18]

IMMUNIZATION DURING THE FOURTH TRIMESTER

Immunization Principles in the Fourth Trimester

Although traditionally considered postpartum care, an imbalance with a focus on antenatal care without a holistic approach to what has been considered postpartum care led to the concept of the fourth trimester.[19] Therefore, assessment of immunization status and review of necessary immunizations is a critical component to this care delivery. The fourth trimester provides an opportunity for promotion of a healthy family with update of vaccinations that could not be administered during pregnancy but also as a catch to ensure immunizations in the interconception period to ensure a subsequent pregnancy can also be healthy. **Table 3** presents the continuum of care and safe administration of immunizations during this interval.[2,20]

Immunization in a Lactating Mother

As a general principle, vaccination with both live attenuated and inactivated vaccines are safe for mother and infant during breastfeeding. This includes MMR and varicella, both of which may have been delayed for nonimmune mothers during pregnancy. Smallpox vaccine is a contraindication for breastfeeding mothers due to a theoretic

Table 2
Indications for pneumococcal vaccination

Type of Pneumococcal Vaccine	Patient's Immune Status	Indications for Vaccine Administration
PCV-13	Immunocompetent	CSF leak Cochlear implant
	Functional or anatomic asplenia	Sickle cell disease Congenital or acquired asplenia
	Immunocompromised	Congenital or acquired immunodeficiency HIV Chronic renal failure Nephrotic syndrome Leukemia Lymphoma Hodgkin disease Generalized malignancy Solid organ transplant Multiple myeloma
PPSV23	Immunocompetent	Chronic heart disease Chronic lung disease Diabetes mellitus CSF leak Cochlear implant Cigarette smoking
	Functional or anatomic asplenia	Sickle cell disease Congenital or acquired asplenia
	Immunocompromised	Congenital or acquired immunodeficiency HIV Chronic renal failure Nephrotic syndrome Leukemia Lymphoma Hodgkin disease Generalized malignancy Solid organ transplant Multiple myeloma

Abbreviations: CSF, cerebrospinal fluid; HIV, human immunodeficiency syndrome; PCV13, 13-valent pneumococcal vaccine; PPSV23, 23-valent pneumococcal polysaccharide vaccine.

Adapted from Centers for Disease Control and Prevention (CDC). Use of 13-valent pneumococcal conjugate vaccine and 23-valent pneumococcal polysaccharide vaccine for adults with immunocompromising conditions: recommendations of the Advisory Committee on Immunization Practices (ACIP). MMWR Morb Mortal Wkly Rep. 2012;61(40):818.

risk of contact transmission to the infant. Yellow fever vaccine is also a precaution and should be avoided in breastfeeding mothers. However, if travel to endemic areas is unavoidable and potential risk of exposure is high, nursing mothers should be vaccinated.[21]

NONROUTINE VACCINATIONS AND VACCINATION CHALLENGES DURING PREGNANCY

Travel During Pregnancy

Travel presents additional considerations for pregnant individuals both for their own risk and potential risk to the fetus. **Table 4** includes select recommendations regarding

Table 3
Recommended vaccinations during pregnancy: preconception to interconception

Time Period	Recommended Vaccines
Preconception care	Human papilloma virus (HPV) vaccine Hepatitis B (HBV) vaccine Measles, mumps, rubella (MMR) vaccine[a] Varicella vaccine Influenza vaccine Diphtheria-tetanus-pertussis vaccine[b]
Antenatal period	Inactivated influenza vaccine Diphtheria-tetanus-pertussis vaccine In specific populations • Hepatitis A vaccine • Hepatitis B vaccine • Meningococcal vaccine • Pneumococcal vaccine (PPSV23)
4th trimester and interconception care	Human papilloma virus (HPV) vaccine Hepatitis A vaccine Hepatitis B (HBV) vaccine Measles, mumps, rubella (MMR) vaccine Varicella vaccine Influenza vaccine Diphtheria-tetanus-pertussis vaccine Meningococcal vaccine Pneumococcal vaccine (PPSV23 and PCV13)

[a] If MMR administered, patient should wait to become pregnant for at least 28 days.
[b] If diphtheria-tetanus-pertussis administered before pregnancy, will need to be repeated at 27 to 36 weeks' gestation.

immunization and vaccine-preventable illnesses in pregnancy. With proper preparation, most pregnant women can travel safely.

Malaria and Pregnancy

Although there is no vaccination against malaria, it is worth mentioning in this section, as malaria acquired during pregnancy, particularly in the case of a primary exposure during a first pregnancy, is associated with poor pregnancy outcomes. It is associated with spontaneous abortion, low birth weight, as well as maternal anemia, and pregnant women are more at risk than nonpregnant women for severe malaria syndromes and death. Malaria also reduces placental transmission of antibodies from mother to fetus, and reduces immune response to vaccination.[22] As no vaccine has been developed, chemoprophylaxis is recommended in the antenatal period for individuals who live in malaria-endemic areas. For those who do not live in endemic areas, travel precaution is advised. If travel is unavoidable, pregnant individuals should take precautions to avoid mosquito bites and should use an antimalarial chemoprophylaxis regimen. Chloroquine should be used in chloroquine-sensitive malaria destination and mefloquine should be used in chloroquine-resistant malaria destinations. Doxycycline (after the fourth month of pregnancy), primaquine, and atovaquone-proguanil should be avoided during pregnancy.[23]

Immunization Considerations During a Measles Outbreak

Measles, also called Rubeola, presents risk to the pregnant mother and the fetus. Maternal risks include pneumonia and increased risk of hospitalization. Measles

Table 4
Special immunization considerations for travel during pregnancy

Disease	Relevant Vaccine and Disease Considerations	
Zika virus[18]	Disease considerations	• Virus is transmitted primarily through the bite of an infected *Aedes* mosquito but can be sexually transmitted as well • Men and women who are planning a pregnancy within the next 3 mo, and individuals who are pregnant, should avoid travel to high-risk areas. • A current list of countries and territories at risk can be found at www.cdc.gov/travel
	Vaccine considerations	There is no available vaccine to date.
Yellow fever[18,23]	Vaccine considerations	• Although most live vaccines are contraindicated, the Advisory Committee on Immunization Practices considers pregnancy a precaution for vaccination and this decision should be individualized. If the risk of exposure is substantial and travel is unavoidable, the risk of exposure may outweigh the risk of the yellow fever vaccine. If the risk of the vaccine is felt to outweigh the risk of exposure, a medical waiver should be issued. • Pregnancy may affect the mounting of an adequate immune response, so serologic testing to confirm immunity is reasonable. • If given during the preconception period, delayed conception for 1 month is advised.
Hepatitis A	Disease considerations	• Hepatitis A has been reported to increase the risk of placental abruption and prematurity.[18]
	Vaccine considerations	• Vaccine safety in pregnancy is not determined. • The decision to vaccine should be based on risk. • The theoretic risk of hepatitis A vaccination is thought to be low.[23]
Japanese encephalitis	Vaccine considerations	• Vaccine safety in pregnancy is not determined.[23]
Rabies[18,23]	Vaccine considerations	• Pregnancy is not a contraindication to preexposure therapy if risk is substantial. • Rabies postexposure prophylaxis should be administered after any high-risk or moderate-risk exposure, including vaccine and immune globulin.
Typhoid fever[30]	Vaccine considerations	• Oral live typhoid vaccine is contraindicated in pregnancy. • Intramuscular vaccine safety in pregnancy is not determined and should be given only if clearly needed.

(continued on next page)

Table 4
(continued)

Disease	Relevant Vaccine and Disease Considerations	
Anthrax[23]	Vaccine considerations	• If the risk of exposure is low, anthrax vaccination is not recommended in pregnant women. • If postexposure prophylaxis is otherwise indicated, it should be given to pregnant women.
Smallpox[23]	Vaccine considerations	• Smallpox vaccine is contraindicated in pregnant women or in women who are trying to conceive. • Pregnant women who have had definite exposure to smallpox (close face-to-face or household proximity with a person infected with smallpox) should be vaccinated.

infection during pregnancy also increases the risk of miscarriage, stillbirth, low birth weight, and preterm delivery. Infants born during an active measles infection are at risk for congenital measles. Infants younger than 12 months are at highest risk of measles-associated morbidity and mortality.[24] Measles cases have recently risen to levels not seen in decades partially due to waning immunization rates in some communities. Any potential contact with measles in a nonimmune pregnant person should be promptly investigated. A nonimmune pregnant person with measles exposure, or with confirmed measles may be a candidate for intravenous immunoglobulin. This decision should be made in consultation with Maternal Fetal Medicine/Perinatology.[25] As noted in previous sections, MMR vaccine is contraindicated in pregnancy. Individuals who are found to be nonimmune to measles or rubella during pregnancy should be vaccinated with MMR as soon as possible after delivery. Infants born to vaccinated mothers typically have immunity lasting until 6 to 9 months of age.[25]

Maternal Immunization in Developing Countries

Maternal immunization may be particularly helpful in developing countries where infant death rates are high often due to infection, attendance at prenatal clinics is high, and breastfeeding is nearly universal. Neonatal tetanus, although still a significant cause of neonatal death, has decreased recently due to immunization with tetanus toxoid during pregnancy.[26] There is some evidence that pneumococcal disease contributes to a significant portion of neonatal deaths before the age at which infants can be vaccinated. Small-scale studies have demonstrated safety of pneumococcal vaccination in pregnant women and pneumococcal antibodies have been shown to cross the placenta and persist for weeks in breastmilk following delivery. More research into the potential for maternal pneumococcal vaccination to reduce neonatal infection and mortality may be warranted.[6,26]

DISCLOSURE

The authors have nothing to disclose.

REFERENCES

1. Betz AG. Immunology: tolerating pregnancy. Nature 2012;490:47–8.

2. Vicari M, Dodet B, Englund J. Protection of newborns through maternal immunization. Vaccine 2003;21(24):3351.
3. Simister NE. Placental transport of immunoglobulin G. Vaccine 2003;21(24):3365–9.
4. Van De Perre P. Transfer of antibody via mother's milk. Vaccine 2003;21(24):3374–6.
5. Ontario Public Health Association. Shift-Enhancing the health of Ontarians: A call to action for preconception health promotion and care 2014. Toronto, ON.
6. World Health Organization. Preconception care: maximizing the gains for maternal and child health [pamphlet]. Geneva (Switzerland): World Health Organization; 2013.
7. Jack BW, Atrash H, Coonrod DV, et al. The clinical content of preconception care: an overview and preparation of this supplement. Obstet Gynecol 2008;199(6 Suppl 2):S266–79.
8. Grohskopf LA, Alyanak E, Broder KR, et al. Prevention and control of seasonal influenza with vaccines: recommendations of the Advisory Committee on Immunization Practices – United States, 2019-20 influenza season. MMWR Recomm Rep 2019;68(No. RR-3):1–21.
9. ACOG Committee on Obstetric Practice. ACOG Committee Opinion No. 732. Influenza vaccination during pregnancy. Obstet Gynecol 2018;131:e109–14.
10. Swamy GK, Heine RP. Vaccinations for pregnant women. Obstet Gynecol 2015;125:212–26.
11. Schillie S, Vellozzi C, Reingold A, et al. Prevention of hepatitis B virus infection in the United States: recommendations of the Advisory Committee on Immunization Practices. MMWR Recomm Rep 2018;67(No. RR-1):1–31.
12. Zolotor AJ, Carlough MC. Update on prenatal care. Am Fam Physician 2014;89(3):199–208.
13. McLean HQ, Parker Fiebelkorn A, Temte JL, et al. Prevention of measles, rubella, congenital rubella syndrome, and mumps, 2013: summary recommendations of the Advisory Committee on Immunization Practices (ACIP). MMWR Recomm Rep 2013;62(RR-04):1–34.
14. American College of Obstetricians and Gynecologists. Update on immunization and pregnancy: tetanus, diphtheria, and pertussis vaccination. Committee Opinion No. 718. Obstet Gynecol 2017;130:e153–7.
15. Fiore AE, Wasley A, Bell BP. Prevention of hepatitis A through active or passive immunization: recommendations of the Advisory Committee on Immunization Practices (ACIP). Advisory Committee on Immunization Practices. MMWR Recomm Rep 2006;55(RR-7):1–23.
16. Viral hepatitis in pregnancy. ACOG Practice Bulletin No. 86. American College of Obstetricians and Gynecologists. Obstet Gynecol 2007;110:941–56.
17. Use of 13-valent pneumococcal conjugate vaccine and 23-valent pneumococcal polysaccharide vaccine for adults with immunocompromising conditions: recommendations of the Advisory Committee on Immunization Practices (ACIP). MMWR Wkly Rep 2012;61(40):816–9.
18. Morof DF, Caroll ID. Pregnant travelers. In: CDC Yellow Book 2020 Chapter 7 Family Travel. Available at: https://wwwnc.cdc.gov/travel/yellowbook/2020/family-travel/pregnant-travelers#5654. Accessed October 6, 2019.
19. Tully KP, Stuebe AM, Verbiest SB. The fourth trimester: a critical transition period with unmet maternal health needs. Obstet Gynecol 2017;217(1):37–41.
20. American College of Obstetricians and Gynecologists. Maternal immunization. ACOG Committee Opinion No. 741. Obstet Gynecol 2018;131:e214–7.

21. Anstey EH, Shealy KR. Travel and breastfeeding. In: CDC Yellow Book 2020 Chapter 7 Family Travel. Available at: https://wwwnc.cdc.gov/travel/yellowbook/2020/family-travel/travel-and-breastfeeding. Accessed October 8, 2019.
22. Duffy PE. Maternal immunization and malaria in pregnancy. Vaccine 2003;21(24):3358–61.
23. ACIP guidelines: guidelines for vaccinating pregnant women. CDC toolkit for prenatal care providers. 2016. Available at: https://www.cdc.gov/vaccines/pregnancy/hcp-toolkit/guidelines.html?CDC_AA_refVal=https%3A%2F%2Fwww.cdc.gov%2Fvaccines%2Fpregnancy%2Fhcp%2Fguidelines.html. Accessed October 6, 2019.
24. Gans H, DeHovitz R, Forghani B, et al. Measles and mumps vaccination as a model to investigate the developing immune system: passive and active immunity during the first year of life. Vaccine 2003;21(24):3398–405.
25. Kachikis A, Oler E, Shree R, et al. Measles and the MMR vaccine: recommendations around pregnancy, including the periconception and postpartum periods. 2019. Available at: http://providerresource.uwmedicine.org/flexpaper/measles-and-the-mmr-vaccine-recommendations-around-pregnancy-including-the-periconception-and-postpartum-periods. Accessed October 6, 2019.
26. Greenwood B. Maternal immunisation in developing countries. Vaccine 2003;21(24):3436–41.
27. Zuo Z, Goel S, Carter JE. Association of cervical cytology and HPV DNA status during pregnancy with placental abnormalities and preterm birth. Am J Clin Pathol 2011;136(2):260–5.
28. Eberhart-Phillips JE, Frederick PD, Baron RC, et al. Measles in pregnancy: a descriptive study of 58 cases. Obstet Gynecol 1993;82:797–801.
29. Siegel M, Fuerst HT. Low birth weight and maternal virus diseases. A prospective study of rubella, measles, mumps, chickenpox, and hepatitis. JAMA 1966;197:680–4.
30. Lo Re V, Gluckman SJ. Travel immunizations. Am Fam Physician 2004;70(1):89–99.

Improving Immunization Coverage in Special Populations

Mary M. Stephens, MD, MPH[a,*], Erin Kavanaugh, MD[b]

KEYWORDS

• Immunization • Vaccination • Health care provider • Chronic disease • Child
• Adolescent • Adult • Screening

KEY POINTS

- Standard immunization schedules include recommendations for patients with chronic diseases. Health care providers should think broadly and also consider the needs of other high-risk populations, such as those with intellectual and neurodevelopmental disabilities and the changing health care status of all their patients, which may change their eligibility for immunization.
- For health care providers, a strategic immunization approach based on age, immunization history, and exposure risk is paramount in maintaining protection and limiting transmission of communicable disease on the front lines of patient care.

INTRODUCTION

Chronic diseases are estimated to affect 45% of the US population and are the leading causes of death and health care expenditures.[1] Immunization is an effective strategy to reduce the burden of suffering and cost of care from chronic disease.

Heart disease, cancer, stroke, chronic obstructive pulmonary disease, and diabetes are the most common chronic diseases, and 25% of adults have 2 or more conditions, with the number of comorbidities increasing with age.[1] In a cohort of adults aged 50 years and older with serious pneumococcal infection who were not immunized for pneumococcal disease, 30-day mortality risk increased based on the number of indications present for immunization by 55% for each indication.[2] Health care providers (HCPs) are a special population worthy of consideration on their own.

[a] Department of Family and Community Medicine, Jefferson University Hospitals, 3 Crescent Drive, Philadelphia, PA 19112, USA; [b] Department of Family and Community Medicine, Family Medicine Residency, Emergency Medicine/Family Medicine Residency, Sidney Kimmel Medical College, Christiana Care Health System, 1401 Foulk Road, Suite 100B, Wilmington, DE 19803, USA
* Corresponding author.
E-mail address: mary.stephens@jefferson.edu

Prim Care Clin Office Pract 47 (2020) 453–465
https://doi.org/10.1016/j.pop.2020.05.002
primarycare.theclinics.com

PATIENTS WITH CHRONIC DISEASES

Standard child and adolescent (ages 18 years or younger) and adult (ages 19 years or older) immunization schedules recommended by the Advisory Committee on Immunization Practices and approved by the Centers for Disease Control and Prevention (CDC) and other major health care organizations identify defined categories of high-risk conditions and chronic diseases (**Table 1**). Individuals with these conditions may be at additional risk and require additional vaccines (or extra doses of vaccines), and live vaccines may be contraindicated in immunosuppressed or otherwise susceptible individuals.[3] Specific situations may require a risk assessment to determine whether the risk posed by a live vaccine is greater than the potential benefit of the vaccine.

Recommended population health strategies to increase immunization rates include addressing access, increasing community demand, and provider-based or system-based interventions (**Table 2**).[7]

Vaccine needs assessment is a critical first step in the process for individual HCPs.[8] The CDC recommends that HCPs assess immunization status at every patient encounter and strongly recommend needed vaccines, regardless of whether the office provides vaccines or not (**Table 3**). Tools exist to help HCPs at the practice/system level. Electronic health care records (EHRs) can be modified to include prompts, and standing orders can be used in systems both with and without EHR capability. Although this strategy may work for straightforward recommendations such as age-based or disease-based recommendations for pneumococcal vaccination, it may still miss immunization recommendations for special situations such as alcoholism or acquired immunocompromising conditions. Standard survey tools exist to help HCPs more easily identify patient-specific factors or special situations that may warrant consideration of additional immunizations.[9,10]

Education aimed at patients with specific chronic conditions may help patients better understand the rationale for immunizations based on disease state and be a time saver for clinicians as well as an opportunity to engage staff in team-based care.[11] Assessment of need for immunizations for chronic diseases is an ongoing process. Clinical indicators in patients change over time based on the activity of their acute and chronic disease states and treatment courses. Contraindications and precautions for vaccine administration are often only temporary and are also subject to change based on new evidence and change in formulation of vaccines. Systems of care and HCPs must incorporate these changes into their counseling practices and workflows.[12] Standard screening questionnaires available from state public health departments and other organizations in multiple languages may facilitate this.[13] Office work flows around EHR prompts should address delaying prompts for a set period of time based on the patient's status rather than indefinitely. For example, with influenza vaccination in a patient presenting with moderate or severe acute illness, the practice alert should be delayed for a uniform time period, such as a week, rather than for the entire influenza season.

ALTERNATIVE SITES FOR IMMUNIZATION

Evidence supports the administration of vaccines during hospitalizations as both safe and effective.[14] The scope of pharmacy-based immunization services (PBISs) varies from state to state but they are an effective way to increase immunization rates for patients with chronic diseases, and evidence suggests that PBISs are accepted by patients.[15] PBISs may be a convenient way for patients to access care after recovery from an acute illness that prevented them from receiving the immunization during

Table 1
Advisory Committee on Immunization Practices vaccination recommendations for immunodeficient individuals

Reason for Altered Vaccine Recommendation	Definition	Contraindicated Vaccines	Recommended Vaccines or Possible Need for Extra Doses	Comments on Effectiveness
HIV/AIDS	Immunosuppression caused by HIV/AIDS	OPV Smallpox BCG LAIV MMRV MMR Varicella Zoster Yellow fever	Pneumococcal Hib HepB	In individuals with mild immunosuppression, MMR and varicella vaccines may be effective. Inactivated vaccines including inactivated influenza may be effective
Malignant neoplasm, transplant, radiation, or immunosuppressive therapy	Patients with cancer with certain types of tumors, organ transplant recipients and those undergoing treatments that suppress immune response should avoid live vaccines but require additional doses of others	All live viral and bacterial vaccines	Pneumococcal Hib	Effectiveness of any vaccine depends on the degree of immunosuppression
Asplenia	Immunodeficiency caused by the absence of spleen function leads to increased risk of certain conditions and can render the live influenza vaccine risky	LAIV	Pneumococcal Meningococcal Hib	Routine vaccines are likely effective
Chronic renal disease	Kidney disease causing immunosuppression or altered immune system function (this is separate from immunosuppressive treatments for renal disease)	LAIV	Pneumococcal HepB	Routine vaccines are likely effective

(*continued on next page*)

Table 1
(continued)

Reason for Altered Vaccine Recommendation	Definition	Contraindicated Vaccines	Recommended Vaccines or Possible Need for Extra Doses	Comments on Effectiveness
Heart disease, history of stroke, chronic lung disease	Individuals with any of these conditions may be at increased risk of complications from influenza and pneumococcal diseases	None	Pneumococcal LAIV	LAIV is contraindicated specifically for children aged 2–4 y with asthma or respiratory difficulty
CSF leaks/cochlear implants	CSF leaks caused by head injury or surgery on the brain or sinuses and surgical implantation of cochlear devices can increase risk of certain infections	LAIV	Pneumococcal	CSF leaks may not require altered immunization practice if they are spinal CSF leaks as opposed to cranial CSF leaks
Chronic liver disease or alcoholism	Damage to the liver can lead to increased susceptibility to pneumococcal and hepatic diseases	LAIV	Pneumococcal HepA	Meningococcal vaccine can be recommended if the individual has any other risk factors. Influenza vaccine is typically recommended but risk of adverse effects must be considered
Diabetes	Diabetes can pose an increased risk for pneumococcal and HepB, and the live influenza vaccine may be contraindicated	LAIV	Pneumococcal HepB	Routine vaccines such as zoster and Tdap may be of increased importance

Abbreviations: AIDS, acquired immunodeficiency syndrome; BCG, bacillus Calmette-Guérin; CSF, cerebrospinal fluid; HepA, hepatitis A; HepB, hepatitis B; Hib, *Haemophilus influenzae* type B; HIV, human immunodeficiency virus; LAIV, live attenuated influenza vaccine; MMRV, measles, mumps, rubella, varicella; MMR, measles, mumps, rubella; OPV, oral polio vaccine; Tdap, tetanus, diphtheria, and pertussis.

Data from Refs.[4–6]

Table 2
Community Preventive Services Task Force findings for increasing vaccination

Intervention	CPSTF Finding
Home visits to increase vaccination rates	Recommended (strong evidence)
Reducing client out-of-pocket costs	Recommended (strong evidence)
Vaccination programs in schools and organized child care centers	Recommended (strong evidence)
Vaccination programs in WIC settings	Recommended (strong evidence)
Client or family incentive rewards	Recommended (strong evidence)
Client reminder and recall systems	Recommended (strong evidence)
Client-held paper immunization records	Insufficient evidence
Clinic-based education when used alone	Insufficient evidence
Community-based interventions implemented in combination	Recommended (strong evidence)
Community-wide education when used alone	Insufficient evidence
Monetary sanction policies	Insufficient evidence
Vaccination requirements for child care, school, and college attendance	Recommended (strong evidence)
Health care system–based interventions implemented in combination	Recommended (strong evidence)
Immunization information systems	Recommended (strong evidence)
Provider assessment and feedback	Recommended (strong evidence)
Provider education when used alone	Insufficient evidence
Provider reminders	Recommended (strong evidence)
Standing orders	Recommended (strong evidence)

Abbreviations: CPSTF, Community Preventive Services Task Force; WIC, Women, Infants, and Children.

From Community Preventive Services Task Force. CPSTF findings for increasing vaccination. The Community Guide. September 1, 2019. Available at: https://www.thecommunityguide.org/content/task-force-findings-increasing-vaccination. Accessed September 12, 2019.

an office visit. In addition, patients may have time to consider educational information shared during an office visit and proceed with immunization on a schedule that is convenient for them without return to the HCP. Public health departments, school-based health centers, and places of employment are other options.

Although a downside to administration outside of the office setting is potential failure to capture and document the immunization in the health record, information-sharing practices and patient education can mitigate this. The CDC currently allows for patient-reported history for select vaccines, such as influenza and pneumococcal vaccination.[16] HCPs should routinely ask patients to provide written documentation of outside immunizations and query them at follow-up visits similarly to what is done with medication reconciliation.

OTHER SPECIAL POPULATIONS/SITUATIONS

Intellectual Disability

Patients with intellectual disabilities (IDs) experience high rates of health disparities and poorer health status, in part because of complex comorbidities as well as challenges with access to care.[17,18] International data show lower rates of vaccination

Table 3
Patient survey to determine recommended vaccinations based on age and situation

Age or Situation	Recommended Vaccines
19 y or older	Seasonal influenza every year Tetanus (Td) every 10 y Single dose of whooping cough (Tdap) Additional dose of Tdap during each pregnancy
60 y or older	Shingles (Zoster) vaccine
65 y or older	Both types of pneumococcal vaccine
Did not receive HPV vaccine series as a child and is any of the following: • Woman 26 y old or younger • man 21 y old or younger • Man aged 22–26 y who has sex with men, has a weakened immune system, or has HIV	HPV vaccine series (3 doses)
Born in the United States after 1956 and does not have immunity against MMR	MMR vaccine
Health care worker	HepB vaccine series MMR vaccine Varicella (chickenpox) vaccine
Has heart disease, asthma, or chronic lung disease	Pneumococcal polysaccharide vaccine
Has type 1 or type 2 diabetes	HepB vaccine series Pneumococcal polysaccharide vaccine
Has a weakened immune system	Both types of pneumococcal vaccine HPV vaccine series if <26 y old and not previously vaccinated Hib vaccine (after hematopoietic stem cell transplant only)
Has HIV	HepB vaccine series Both types of pneumococcal vaccine HPV vaccine series if <26 y old and not previously vaccinated
Has chronic liver disease	Hepatitis A vaccine series HepB vaccine series Pneumococcal polysaccharide vaccine
Does not have a spleen, or spleen does not work well	Hib vaccine Meningococcal vaccine Both types of pneumococcal vaccines
Man who has sex with men	Hepatitis A vaccine series HepB vaccine series HPV vaccine series (if 26 y of age or younger and not previously vaccinated)
Laboratory worker who may be exposed to isolates of *Neisseria meningitidis* or specimens containing hepatitis A or B virus	Hepatitis A vaccine series HepB vaccine series Meningococcal vaccine

(continued on next page)

Table 3
(*continued*)

Age or Situation	Recommended Vaccines
College freshman living in a residence hall	Meningococcal vaccine MMR vaccine
Planning to travel outside the United States	Varies depending on travel destination

Abbreviations: HPV, human papilloma virus; Td, tetanus and diphtheria.
From Centers for Disease Control and Prevention. Healthcare provider office information. February 2015. Available at: https://www.cdc.gov/vaccines/hcp/adults/downloads/patient-intake-form.pdf. Accessed September 19, 2019.

for children with ID compared with the general population for nearly all vaccinations at all ages.[19–21] As in the general population, a survey or health review tool may increase rates of immunization.[22]

Neurologic or Neurodevelopmental Disabilities

Although not identified on standard immunization grids as a high-risk group, the Advisory Committee on Immunization Practices has recognized children with neurologic or neurodevelopmental disabilities as a high-risk group for complications of influenza since 2005.[23] A survey of primary care and specialty physicians providing care to high-risk children showed significant knowledge gaps in recognition of high-risk conditions, with only 46% of physicians recognizing ID as a high-risk condition.[23] Other high-risk conditions include epilepsy, cerebral palsy, stroke, spinal cord injury, and other brain conditions. Children with neurodevelopmental disabilities are at increased risk of new-onset seizures, intensive care admission, and mechanical ventilation compared with children without neurodevelopmental disabilities but with other high-risk conditions.[24] Of note, although a significant percentage of parents of patients in the high-risk group refused vaccines because of safety and effectiveness concerns in a parental survey, 7% declined because the vaccine was not recommended by the physician.[23]

Human Papilloma Virus Vaccination and Intellectual Disability

Data from the United Kingdom show that human papilloma virus (HPV) immunization rates are lower in girls with moderate or severe intellectual disabilities.[25] Although there is limited research about rates of cervical cancer in this population, there is evidence that people with mild ID have rates of sexual activity comparable with the general population and a significant percentage with moderate (32%) and severe ID (9%) engage in sexual activity.[26] Limited data also indicate that rates of screening for cervical cancer are much lower in women with ID compared with the general population, potentially increasing the risk associated with cervical cancer.[25] In addition, women with ID are significantly more likely to experience sexual abuse than the general population.[26] Strategies to improve rates of HPV vaccination include provider and parental education about risks and patient-centered, developmentally appropriate counseling for patients with standard HCP recommendations for HPV immunization.[25]

Down Syndrome

The incidence of Down syndrome (DS) is 1 per 750 live births, and it is the most common genetic cause of ID. In recent years, research has shown that people with DS have significant defects in T-cell and B-cell function creating a relatively immunocompromised state and are at increased risk for death from sepsis and pneumonia.[27,28] In

Table 4
Centers for Disease Control and Prevention and Advisory Committee on Immunization Practices vaccination recommendations for health care providers

Vaccination	Evidence-Based Recommendation for Health Care Providers	Route of Vaccination
HepB	If no evidence of (1) immunization or (2) prior immunity, recommend 2-dose or 3-dose series with follow-up confirmatory serologic testing	IM[42]
Influenza	Recommended annually • If vaccine supply is limited, HCPs are in the category of recommended to receive[43]	IM (or intranasally)[42]
MMR	Measles and Mumps: 2 doses of MMR vaccination recommended if: • Born 1957 or after and have not been vaccinated • Do not have blood work showing serologic immunity Rubella: 1 dose of MMR vaccine recommended if: • Born 1957 or after and have not been vaccinated • Do not have blood work showing serologic immunity • *May eventually get 2 doses because of the combined nature of the vaccine The simplest approach to any concern regarding immunization status or documentation of MMR is to revaccinate regardless of setting[44]	Subcut[42]
Varicella	2 doses recommend, 4 wk apart, if: • An HCP who has not had chickenpox • An HCP who has not had varicella vaccination Do not have blood work showing serologic immunity	Subcut[42]
Tdap	If not received Tdap previously, a 1-time dose is recommended, regardless of when received Td Recommend Td boosters every 10 y after Tdap	IM[42]
Meningococcus	Recommend 1-time dose if routinely exposed	IM[42]
Hepatitis A	Not occupationally acquired; not recommended to screen or vaccinate HCPs[6,7] In the event of an outbreak, discuss options with Employee Health Department	—

Abbreviation: IM, intramuscular.

multivariate analysis, respiratory failure was the sole risk factor for mortality in patients with DS compared with the general population, with a greater than 9 times relative risk of death.[29] Declining levels of antibody protection against hepatitis B have also been shown.[30]

For these reasons, specialty organizations and clinics serving patients with DS have made recommendations to consider immunizing patients with DS according to recommendations for patients who are immunocompromised or have a chronic lung condition.[31–33] In addition, consideration should be given to checking antibody levels or giving a booster dose of hepatitis B vaccine for individuals with DS at high risk of disease because of evidence of waning immunity.[30]

Autism

Approximately 1% to 2% of the population has autism spectrum disorder (ASD).[34] Individuals with autism are at increased risk for chronic disease, unintentional injury, medication-related side effects, and early mortality.[35] Medical comorbidities, including ID and seizure disorders, are associated with premature death. Complex issues such as behavioral problems and limited ability to perform activities of daily living may also contribute to early mortality.[35] In part because of disproven historical concerns about links between immunization and autism, children with ASD and their younger siblings are still undervaccinated compared with the general population.[36] Teens and adults with ASD may be at risk for vaccine-preventable disease because of parental refusal of vaccination during childhood. Tools and strategies are available to help HCPs counsel patients with ASD, and their families or caregivers when appropriate, about recommended immunizations and close care gaps.[37–39]

HEALTH CARE PROVIDERS

HCPs represent a special population of their own. HCPs are routinely potentially exposed to communicable and deadly diseases, and must be maximally protected via vaccination as a means of preventing illness.[40] Most organizations require immunization or proof of immunity status on hiring. HCPs are at risk not only for acquisition of disease but for potentiating transmission if not adequately immunized.[41] Specifically, HCPs should expect to consider vaccination for hepatitis B; influenza; measles, mumps and rubella; varicella; tetanus; diphtheria; pertussis; and meningococcus. **Table 4** reviews high-level recommendations for HCPs.[40,41]

SUMMARY

The strongest predictor of patients receiving recommended vaccines is whether HCPs recommend the vaccine.[45] Providers need to be aware of current recommendations and develop team-based strategies for assessment and workflow in their offices to improve vaccination rates for patients with chronic disease. HCPs need to be aware of their own immune status and up to date on evidence-based recommendations to protect both themselves and their patients from preventable transmission of communicable diseases.

A Case Example

EN is a 23-year-old woman with DS, seizure disorder, and hypothyroidism. She presents for a new patient visit in October with her older sister, who is an established patient in your practice. Her sister asks what recommendations you have to help keep EN healthy. She has only recently moved in with her sister because her parents are no longer able to care for her because of their own chronic health issues. EN works in a coffee shop 20 hours a week, volunteers at the DS clinic at the local children's hospital, exercises regularly, and is involved in Special Olympics. Her sister has no idea about her immunization history. She knows she has not received any immunizations since she moved in with her 6 months ago.

It is October so you make a strong recommendation that both sisters get their flu shots today. The patient is able to communicate that she is nervous because she cannot remember the last time she had a shot. Your medical assistant (MA) describes the procedure to her using plain language and offers to give her older sister the flu shot first so that she understands better what a shot involves. When she understands that getting a flu shot is no harder than getting her blood drawn, she feels much better. She knows she is good at that. The sister agrees and puts on EN's favorite play list on her phone to help her relax and promises her they will do something fun after the visit like they did the last time she had blood drawn. Both young women get their flu shots without a problem, and the patient signs a release of medical information to obtain vaccination records from her former pediatrician.

Your MA asks you to review the records when they arrive and you give the patient and her sister a call to review your recommendations. You let them know EN is up to date on her tetanus, diphtheria, and pertussis (Tdap) and had titers drawn for immunity to hepatitis B when she started volunteering at the children's hospital 3 years ago. You give a strong recommendation for the HPV series, as is your usual practice. The older sister received the vaccine, and she encourages EN to get it. You make a recommendation for pneumococcal vaccination (pneumococcal polysaccharide vaccine) because the patient has DS and this is a common practice recommended by DS specialty organizations given the additional health risks people with DS face.

EN and her sister agree to make a nurse visit for the first HPV shot and the pneumococcal vaccine. EN tells you she has been working hard on eating healthier since she saw you last and asks whether she can get her weight checked at the visit. You agree and place orders in your EHR for the HPV series and pneumococcal vaccination. Your MA administers the vaccines without difficulty and sets up a follow-up nurse visit for the second HPV shot on a day the patient and her sister are both off from work. She will receive her third HPV shot when she sees you for her 6-month follow-up visit. She asks the MA to let you know she has lost 0.9 kg (2 pounds) since she gave up sugar-sweetened beverages.

ACKNOWLEDGMENTS

The authors thank Wendy Ross, MD, FAAP and Alexander Fossi, MPH from the Jefferson Center for Autism and Neurodiversity for their assistance with article preparation.

DISCLOSURE

The authors have nothing to disclose.

REFERENCES

1. Raghupathi W, Raghupathi V. An Empirical Study of Chronic Diseases in the United States: A Visual Analytics Approach to Public Health. Int J Environ Res Public Health 2018;15(3):E431.
2. Morton J, Morrill H, LaPlante K, et al. Risk stacking of pneumococcal vaccination indications increases mortality in unvaccinated adults with Streptococcus pneumoniae infections. Vaccine 2017;35(13):1692–7.

3. Advisory Committee on Immunization Practices. Contraindications and Precautions. General Best Practice Guidelines for Immunization: Best Practices Guidance of the Advisory Committee on Immunization Practices (ACIP). 2019. Available at: https://www.cdc.gov/vaccines/hcp/acip-recs/general-recs/contraindications.html. Accessed September 19, 2019.
4. Advisory Committee on Immunization Practices. Altered Immunocompetence. Vaccine Recommendations and Guidelines of the ACIP. 2019. Available at: https://www.cdc.gov/vaccines/hcp/acip-recs/general-recs/immunocompetence.html. Accessed September 19, 2019.
5. Centers for Disease Control and Prevention. Vaccines Indicated for Adults Based on Medical Indications. Immunization Schedules. 2019. Available at: https://www.cdc.gov/vaccines/schedules/hcp/imz/adult-conditions.html. Accessed September 19, 2019.
6. Centers for Disease Control and Prevention. Vaccines Indicated for Persons Aged 0 through 18 years Based on Medical Indications. Immunization Schedules. 2019. Available at: https://www.cdc.gov/vaccines/schedules/hcp/imz/child-indications.html. Accessed September 19, 2019.
7. Community Preventive Services Task Force. CPSTF Findings for Increasing Vaccination. The Community Guide. 2019. Available at: https://www.thecommunityguide.org/content/task-force-findings-increasing-vaccination. Accessed September 12, 2019.
8. Centers for Disease Control and Prevention. Vaccine Needs Assessment. Centers for Disease Control and Prevention. 2016. Available at: https://www.cdc.gov/vaccines/hcp/adults/downloads/standards-immz-practice-assessment.pdf. Accessed September 12, 2019.
9. Centers for Disease Control and Prevention. Healthcare Provider Office Information. Centers for Disease Control and Prevention. 2015. Available at: https://www.cdc.gov/vaccines/hcp/adults/downloads/patient-intake-form.pdf. Accessed September 19, 2019.
10. Immunization Action Coalition. Which Vaccines Do I Need Today? Immunize.org. 2019. Available at: https://www.immunize.org/catg.d/p4036.pdf. Accessed September 19, 2019.
11. Centers for Disease Control and Prevention. Adults with Chronic Health Conditions. Adult Vaccination Resources. 2016. Available at: https://www.cdc.gov/vaccines/hcp/adults/for-patients/health-conditions.html. Accessed September 19, 2019.
12. Ezeanolue E, Harriman K, Hunter P, et al. Best Practices Guidance of the Advisory Committee on Immunization Practices (ACIP). General Best Practice Guidelines for Immunization. Available at: www.cdc.gov/vaccines/hcp/acip-recs/general-recs/downloads/general-recs.pdf. Accessed September 12, 2019.
13. Immunization Action Coalition. Handouts: Topic Index. Immunize.org. September 9, 2019. Available at: https://www.immunize.org/handouts/screening-vaccines.asp. Accessed September 19, 2019.
14. Tartof S, Qian L, Liu I, et al. Safety of Influenza Vaccination Administered During Hospitalization. Mayo Clin Proc 2019;94(3):397–407.
15. Burson R, Buttenheim A, Armstrong A, et al. Community pharmacies as sites of adult vaccination: A systematic review. Hum Vaccin Immunother 2016;12(12):3146–59.
16. Immunization Action Coalition. Documenting Vaccination. Immunize.org. 2019. Available at: https://www.immunize.org/askexperts/documenting-vaccination.asp. Accessed September 1, 2019.

17. Brameld K, Spilsbury K, Rosenwax L, et al. Use of health services in the last year of life and cause of death in people with intellectual disability: a retrospective matched cohort study. BMJ Open 2018;8(2):e020268.
18. Krahn G, Hammond L, Turner A. A cascade of disparities: health and health care access for people with intellectual disabilities. Ment Retard Dev Disabil Res Rev 2006;12(1):70–82.
19. Emerson E, Robertson J, Baines S, et al. Vaccine Coverage among Children with and without Intellectual Disabilities in the UK: Cross Sectional Study. BMC Public Health 2019;19(1):748.
20. Lin JD, Lin PY, Lin LP. Universal hepatitis B vaccination coverage in children and adolescents with intellectual disabilities. Res Dev Disabil 2010;31(2):338–44.
21. Yen CF, Lin JD. Factors influencing administration of hepatitis B vaccine to community-dwelling teenagers aged 12–18 with an intellectual disability. Res Dev Disabil 2011;32(6):2943–9.
22. Lennox N, Bain C, Rey-Conde T, et al. Cluster Randomized-Controlled Trial of Interventions to Improve Health for Adults with Intellectual Disability Who Live in Private Dwellings. J Appl Res Intellect Disabil 2010;23(4):303–11.
23. Smith M, Peacock G, Uyeki T, et al. Influenza vaccination in children with neurologic or neurodevelopmental disorders. Vaccine 2015;33(20):2322–7.
24. Burton C, Vaudry W, Moore D, et al. Burden of Seasonal Influenza in Children With Neurodevelopmental Conditions. Pediatr Infect Dis J 2014;33(7):710–4.
25. MacLeod R, Tuffrey C. Immunisation against HPV in girls with intellectual disabilities. Arch Dis Child 2014;99(12):1068–70.
26. Servais L. Sexual health care in persons with intellectual disabilities. Ment Retard Dev Disabil Res Rev 2006;12(1):48–56.
27. Intrinsic defect of the immune system in children with Down syndrome: a review. In: Kusters M, Verstegen R, Gemen E, et al, editors. Clin Exp Immunol 2009; 156(2):189–93.
28. Huggard D, Molloy E. Do children with Down syndrome benefit from extra vaccinations? Arch Dis Child 2018;103(11):1085–7.
29. Uppal H, Chandran S, Potluri R. Risk factors for mortality in Down syndrome. J Intellect Disabil Res 2015;59(9):873–81.
30. Eijsvoogel N, Hollegien M, Bok V, et al. Declining antibody levels after hepatitis B vaccination in Down syndrome: A need for booster vaccination? J Med Virol 2017; 89(9):1682–5.
31. Marder L. Immunisation. Down's Syndrome Association. 2019. Available at: https://www.downs-syndrome.org.uk/?wpdmdl=6987&ind=0. Accessed September 13, 2019.
32. Adult Down Syndrome Center. Pneumonia vaccine recommendation. Advocate Medical Group; 2014.
33. Ramos E. Important Vaccines to Consider for People with Down Syndrome. Massachusetts General Hospital. 2017. Available at: https://www.massgeneral.org/children/down-syndrome/vaccines-to-consider.aspx. Accessed September 13, 2019.
34. Centers for Disease Control and Prevention. Autism Spectrum Disorder (ASD). Centers for Disease Control and Prevention. 2019. Available at: https://www.cdc.gov/ncbddd/autism/data.html. Accessed September 21, 2019.
35. DaWalt LS, Hong J, Greenberg J, et al. Mortality in individuals with autism spectrum disorder: Predictors over a 20-year period. Autism 2019;23(7):1732–9.

36. Zerbo O, Modaressi S, Goddard K, et al. Vaccination Patterns in Children After Autism Spectrum Disorder Diagnosis and in Their Younger Siblings. JAMA Pediatr 2018;172(5):469–75.
37. Centers for Disease Control and Prevention. Provider Resources for Vaccine Conversations with Parents. Resources for Professionals. 2016. Available at: https://www.cdc.gov/vaccines/partners/childhood/professionals.html. Accessed September 21, 2019.
38. Centers for Disease Control and Prevention. Provider Resources for Vaccine Conversations with Parents. Centers for Disease Control and Prevention. 2015. Available at: https://www.cdc.gov/vaccines/hcp/conversations/index.html. Accessed September 19, 2019.
39. Immunization Action Coalition. Autism. Immunize.org. 2019. Available at: https://www.immunize.org/autism/. Accessed September 21, 2019.
40. Centers for Disease Control and Prevention. Healthcare Workers. Vaccine Information for Adults. 2016. Available at: https://www.cdc.gov/vaccines/adults/rec-vac/hcw.html. Accessed September 19, 2019.
41. Advisory Committee on Immunization Practices. Immunization of Health-Care Personnel: Recommendations of the Advisory Committee on Immunization Practices (ACIP). MMWR Recomm Rep 2011;60(RR-7):1 45. Available at: https://www.cdc.gov/mmwr/preview/mmwrhtml/rr6007a1.htm. Accessed September 19, 2019.
42. Immunization Action Coalition. Healthcare Personnel Vaccination Recommendations. Immunize.org. 2017. Available at: https://www.immunize.org/catg.d/p2017.pdf. Accessed September 19, 2019.
43. Advisory Committee on Immunization Practices. Prevention and Control of seasonal influenza with vaccines: recommendations of the Advisory Committee on immunization practices (ACIP)—United States, 2019-20. Centers for Disease Control & Prevention; 2019. Available at: https://www.cdc.gov/flu/professionals/acip/summary/summary-recommendations.htm. Accessed September 19, 2019.
44. Advisory Committee on Immunization Practices. General best practice guidelines for immunization: best practices guidance of the advisory committee on immunization practices (ACIP). Centers for Disease Control and Prevention; 2017. Available at: https://www.cdc.gov/vaccines/hcp/acip-recs/general-recs/special-situations.html. Accessed September 19, 2019.
45. Johnson D, Nichol K, Lipczynski K. Barriers to Adult Immunization. Am J Med 2008;121:528–35.

Recognizing Vaccine-Preventable Diseases and Managing Outbreaks

Jennifer L. Hamilton, MD, PhD

KEYWORDS

- Disease surveillance • Disease outbreaks • Measles • Mumps
- Meningococcal infection • Hepatitis A • Pertussis

KEY POINTS

- Cases of vaccine-preventable diseases may be difficult to recognize, because clinicians may not have encountered these illnesses previously.
- Outbreaks may be associated with low levels of vaccination, with high levels of vaccination but with decreasing immunity, with travel destinations and transportation hubs, and with dense populations.
- Familiarity with distinct risks of local populations and with diagnostic findings for vaccine-preventable diseases will help clinicians recognize these infections.
- If vaccine-preventable disease is suspected, close coordination with local health department officials is vital for patient care and population health.

INTRODUCTION

Although movies and television shows might suggest that a disease outbreak necessarily involves a rapidly spreading novel infection with high morbidity and mortality, outbreaks are more generally defined as the occurrence of a disease beyond what would be expected for a particular area, population, or time. Some outbreaks are predictable, as when influenza becomes epidemic during most winters. This article addresses outbreaks of vaccine preventable illnesses that generally have low incidence rates. Two related factors intertwine to add to the challenge of managing outbreaks: as more parents decide not to vaccinate their children, the risk of disease outbreaks increases; and because effective immunizations for many illnesses were introduced over 40 years ago, younger clinicians may not have ever seen a case of once-common infections. Therefore, this article

Department of Family, Community, and Preventive Medicine, Drexel University College of Medicine, 10 Shurs Lane, Suite 301, Philadelphia, PA 19127, USA
E-mail address: jlh88@drexel.edu
Twitter: @jeneralist1 (J.L.H.)

Prim Care Clin Office Pract 47 (2020) 467–481
https://doi.org/10.1016/j.pop.2020.05.003
0095-4543/20/

- Reviews the link between vaccination rates and outbreak risk
- Describes other factors that make a community more likely to experience an outbreak
- Discusses how to notify public health officials in response to patients' clinical presentation and laboratory results
- Summarizes key diagnostic findings for diseases that have been involved in recent US outbreaks, along with recommendations for laboratory testing, initial treatment, and care for contacts.

RISK OF OUTBREAK

The ability to recognize the first case of a disease within a given area becomes more important in locales that are at higher risk of an outbreak. Low vaccination rates, of course, are one key risk factor. The threshold vaccination rate at which sustained transmission of disease is possible varies for different illnesses. An illness that has a long period of transmissibility before symptoms develop may spread more widely than one for which severe symptoms develop early; a disease that is spread by casual contact or airborne particles will likely infect more people than one spread through close contact, blood, or stool.

For vaccination to produce community protection (herd immunity), enough people must be immune that a contagious person transmits the infection to less than one vulnerable person. Measles is often the outbreak disease that first appears in an undervaccinated community. Because one person with measles can spread the disease to 12 to 18 others, somewhere between 11/12 and 17/18 of the population—92% to 94%—must be immune to maintain community protection.

Undervaccinated persons are not evenly distributed geographically. Communities with low vaccination rates develop, perhaps because of poor access to immunizations or because of shared health beliefs. Thus, even if a county or state has high vaccination rates overall, at-risk communities may exist. Public schools in a state without religious/philosophic objection exemptions can be expected to have higher vaccination rates than a private school affiliated with a group that shuns medical interventions. (However, be mindful that low vaccination rates among members of a group may arise from limited access to care, rather than from shared health care beliefs, even when the group is identified by religion.[1])

Low rates of immunity create fertile ground for outbreaks; travelers often bring in the first case. Locations with many travelers, such as those close to a major airport, have increased risks. Communities with close ties to other areas experiencing outbreaks may also be concerns. Examples of outbreaks with identified relationships to international travel include US measles cases in 2014 associated with travel to the Philippines and the 2018/19 outbreak of measles in New York communities with close ties to Israel. The measles outbreak centered at Disneyland in California in 2014 to 2015 was similarly associated with international and domestic travel. This suggests that clinicians near high-travel sites who familiarize themselves with local vaccination coverage patterns can be aware of their higher risks and better prepare themselves to identify and respond to cases of vaccine-preventable diseases. To that end, many states publish rates of childhood vaccination or nonmedical exemptions at the level of counties/parishes or individual school districts.[2]

Not all outbreaks, however, can fit this model. Outbreaks can also occur in highly vaccinated populations if the population is dense enough and immunity for some has waned over time; this can be seen in outbreaks of mumps centered at colleges and universities. Persons who have been vaccinated may nonetheless be susceptible to illness: immunity generally wanes over time, and some persons never develop primary immunity from vaccination. As another example, some vaccines against disease caused by *Neisseria meningitidis* may not prevent asymptomatic carriage of bacteria.[3] The virulent form of *N meningitidis* does not need to be introduced to a community from outside; but once the transformation occurs, it can be spread by close contact. Evidence suggests that asymptomatic, vaccinated persons can transmit lethal strains to others through close contact.[4]

Putting these lines of reasoning together, clinicians who want to be better able to identify initial cases of disease outbreaks can

- Be aware of local vaccination rates, noting possible pockets of lower rates
- Monitor outbreak reports (www.cdc.gov/outbreaks)
- Know history and examination findings for illnesses that may be seen in an outbreak

WORKING WITH LOCAL/REGIONAL HEALTH DEPARTMENT

The diagnosis of an illness that may mark the beginning of an outbreak is a necessary, but limited, step in managing the outbreak. Measles, mumps, rubella, pertussis, meningococcal infections, hepatitis A and B, and many other vaccine-preventable diseases should be reported to local health departments and to the Centers for Disease Control and Prevention (For a list of nationally notifiable diseases, see https://wwwn.cdc.gov/nndss/conditions/). Some local jurisdictions require reports directly from clinicians. Clinicians provide information necessary to outbreak investigation that simply cannot be obtained from laboratory results alone. For example, measles infectivity ranges from 4 days before, although 4 days after rash appears; knowing when the rash appeared is a key piece of information. Also note that verbal notification by phone may be required within 24 hours of when the diagnosis is suspected, not confirmed.

For a busy clinician evaluating a patient who may have a rarely seen illness, mandated reporting may function as a free consult with a public health staff member who might have followed-up on this disease multiple times in the past and may be very familiar with what tests need to be done. Public health staff can also help track down difficult-to-contact patients.

Because early consultation with public health officials is such a vital part of outbreak management, the reader is encouraged to look up appropriate phone numbers in advance of needing them and record them somewhere they can be readily accessed later, such as in the contact list on a smartphone. The National Association of County and City Health Officials maintains a searchable list of local health departments at https://www.naccho.org/membership/lhd-directory.

Be prepared to share the following key information with public health personnel:[5,6]

- Patient demographics: name, address, date of birth, sex, ethnicity/race, place of birth, local resident versus visitor
- Date of symptom onset and symptoms displayed
- Vaccination status
- Risk factors
- Travel history (not just where the patient could have gotten sick but also where have they been since then)
- Occupation
- Known contacts

Diagnostic details, appropriate laboratory work, timeframes for follow-up, and isolation requirements vary among these illnesses. The following summary charts address

Table 1
Measles

Peak ages	• In the prevaccination era, measles was largely a disease of children (preschool or young school age).[8] • Cases reported to the CDC from January 1—April 26 2019 had median age of 5 y, with 24% of cases aged 20 years or older.[9]
Key findings on presentation	• Clinical case definition: generalized rash lasting 3 or more days; temp 101.0 or higher; cough, coryza, or conjunctivitis.[5] • Rash starts 2–4 d after fever, beginning on the face/head, then down to the trunk and extremities.[10] • Koplik spots occur in about 70% of cases, appearing 1–2 d before rash onset.[10] • Travel history, contact with travelers, and vaccination status can support the diagnosis. • If clinical suspicion is high, do not wait for 3 d of rash (to satisfy case definition) before taking action.
Incubation and infection timing	• Approximately 8–12 d from infection until fever; rash generally appears 4 d later.[7,8] • Most patients are contagious from 4 d before the rash appears until 4 d after. Immunocompromised patients may remain contagious for the full duration of their illness.[8]
Differential includes	• Febrile illnesses with rash: parvovirus, scarlet fever, dengue, Kawasaki.[7,10] • Rubella may also be considered if there is no history of MMR vaccine but tests for measles are negative.[7,10]
Laboratories	• Measles IgM is most commonly used for diagnosis.[5,10,11] IgM collected within 72 h of rash onset has a 23% chance of yielding a false-negative result.[5,10] Immunized persons may not spike IgM, so PCR is more important in this group. • Note that measles continues to be rare enough that the risk of false-positive IgM results is significant; the positive predictive value (PPV) of the test is low. Try to restrict testing to likely cases with identified risk factors.[5] • IgG seroconversion can also be used.[5] This test, too, has a low PPV. Can expect IgG seroconversion in 7–10 d after onset of rash in unvaccinated persons. • Measles RNA RT-PCR, using throat swab, nasopharyngeal swab, or (with lower yield) urine. PCR testing enables genotyping in outbreaks.[10] • "Efforts should be made to obtain a serum sample and throat swab (or nasopharyngeal swab) from suspected cases at first contact"[5] • May also consider testing for group A streptococcus to evaluate for scarlet fever
If you suspect your patient has measles	• Contact health department immediately. Do not wait for laboratory results. • Isolate patient: "case patients should be isolated for 4 d after rash onset"[5] • Evaluate for other at-risk persons: patient contacts who may be un- or undervaccinated, immunocompromised, pregnant, etc.

(continued on next page)

Table 1 (*continued*)	
Care of contacts	• There is limited information on efficacy of MMR and Ig postexposure for disease prevention.[5] Those at high risk of severe disease (eg, younger than 12 mo, pregnant without evidence of immunity, severely immunocompromised) should receive IG. Contact your health department to arrange IG delivery. • Vaccination within 72 h of exposure should be considered for all incompletely vaccinated persons.[8] Although vaccination is generally recommended starting at age 12 mo, MMR vaccine has been given to children as young as 6 mo of age with good efficacy in prior US measles outbreaks.[8]
Guidelines for school, day care, college, etc.	• Isolated cases may return fifth day after rash onset if not immunocompromised.[5]
In health care settings	• For those diagnosed with measles, standard precautions plus airborne precautions (negative air pressure) until 4 d after the onset of the rash.[8] Patients should be asked to wear a mask.[5] • "Exposed susceptible patients should be placed on airborne precautions from day 5 after the first exposure until day 21 after last exposure."[8]

Abbreviations: IgM, immunoglobulin M; MMR, measles, mumps, and rubella; RT-PCR, real-time polymerase chain reaction.

key features of measles, mumps, invasive meningococcal disease, hepatitis A, and pertussis.

MEASLES

Measles is a highly contagious illness: one person can infect 12 to 18 others. Therefore, a community needs to have more than 93% of persons immune to prevent an outbreak. Measles transmission may be the first sign of an underimmunized community. Before the widespread use of vaccination this disease was responsible for more than 2 million annual deaths worldwide[7] (**Table 1**).

MUMPS

Mumps outbreaks have occurred in college and university populations in which greater than 96% of students have received 2 doses of vaccine.[12] The recommended 2 doses may produce immunity in only 88% of recipients.[13,14] Further, immunity wanes with time: in one outbreak, students who received their second measles, mumps, and rubella (MMR) vaccine more than 13 years before the outbreak had 9 times the risk of infection than those who had second dose within 2 years.[12] Those who develop clinical illness after 2 doses of vaccine have a reduced risk of hospitalization, orchitis, and meningitis[15] (**Table 2**).

Outbreaks have also occurred in communities other than educational institutions: recent examples include the Marshallese communities in Arkansas, Hawaii, Washington, and Colorado.[16] An outbreak in Alaska led to a third dose of MMR vaccine being recommended statewide.[17]

Table 2
Mumps

Peak ages	• Mumps had been disease of childhood, with peak incidence in children aged 5–9 y[18] • Now outbreaks occur in close-knit communities or universities. From January 2016–June 2017, "most cases occurred in young adults" (median age 21 y),[19] but a 2009–2010 outbreak in Guam had median age 12 y (range 2 mo–79 y)[14]
Key findings on presentation	• Parotitis, unilateral or bilateral • "Low-grade" fever is common[14] • Chills, headache, and "slight increase in temperature" may occur about 24 h before onset of parotid swelling[18] • *Vaccination history may not be reassuring:* in US outbreaks from January 2016–June 2017, "among the 7187 of 9200 patients with known vaccination status, 70% had received 2 doses of MMR vaccine"[19]
Incubation and infection timing	• Incubation is generally 16–18 d; observed range 12–25 d after exposure[14,20] • Contagious from several days before parotitis starts through 5 d after[20]
Differential includes	• Epstein-Barr virus (EBV), influenza, parvovirus B19, Coxsackie A virus, sialolithiasis[14,18] • In one case series, 5.7% of suspect cases were positive for mumps; 19.8% were EBV[18]
Laboratories	• Serum IgM may be negative, especially if patient had been previously vaccinated. It is difficult to identify an IgG increase, because IgG may be elevated at the time of initial draw • RT-PCR yield may be low if collected more than 3 d after onset of parotitis • It may be difficult to rule out mumps by negative laboratory results • When obtaining RT-PCR, can obtain swab samples from parotid duct, other salivary gland ducts, and throat. If the patient presents with orchitis, may use urine samples[14] • EBV testing may also be helpful
If you suspect your patient has mumps	• Isolate the patient with droplet precautions for 5 d after the onset of parotitis[14] • Notify health department
Care of contacts	• Immune globulin is not effective as postexposure prophylaxis. Mumps vaccination has not been shown to be effective if administered after exposure. However, vaccination may be offered to protect against *later* exposures[20]
Guidelines for school, day care, college, etc.	• During outbreaks, a third dose of MMR vaccine is recommended[19] • Exclusion of susceptible persons during outbreaks until the 26th day after parotitis onset in the last person with mumps at the affected institutions may decrease risk of infection. "Excluded students can be readmitted immediately after they are vaccinated"[14]
In health care settings	• Isolate the patient if mumps is suspected; use droplet precautions in addition to standard precautions. Maintain isolation until 5 d after parotid swelling began[20] • "Health care personnel with mumps illness should be excluded for 5 d after the onset of parotitis"[14]

MENINGOCOCCAL DISEASE

Recall that in invasive meningococcal disease (IMD), death can occur within hours of onset of symptoms. The overall case-fatality rate in the United States is approximately 15%. Up to a fifth of survivors face sequelae such as amputations, hearing loss, and neurologic disabilities.[21] If clinical suspicion of meningococcal disease exists, early action is vital (**Table 3**).

Persons with asplenia or complement deficiencies are at much higher risk of IMD. Medications that act as complement inhibitors, such as eculizumab (Solaris) or ravulizumab (Ultomiris) may have more than 1000 times the usual risk for getting meningococcal disease.[22] Vaccinated persons taking complement inhibitors have developed IMD.

A prospective study of US high school students found carriage rates of 3.2% to 4.1%.[23] Historical data have carriage at 10% of adults.[24] Vaccination may not protect against carriage and transmission of invasive strains.[25]

Less than 5% of cases are associated with identified outbreaks.[21] When identified outbreaks occur, incidence rates are lower than for many other diseases. An outbreak of 9 cases may develop over the course of a year,[26] making it difficult to delineate the end of the crisis.

HEPATITIS A

Recall that hepatitis A virus (HAV) spreads via fecal-oral transmission. An outbreak can be associated with contaminated food or with fecally contaminated environments. Small-scale food-related transmission may be traced to a particular food handler at a local restaurant, but large-scale food-related HAV can span continents, as in a Scandinavian outbreak linked to strawberries from Egypt and Morocco.[34] HAV is also associated with person-to-person transmission among homeless populations and users of illicit drugs, as in 2017/18 in San Diego[35] and in 2019 in Philadelphia[36] (**Table 4**).

Hepatitis A vaccination was not recommended for most US children until 2006. The vaccine is now also recommended for those experiencing homelessness,[37] but this may be difficult to implement.

PERTUSSIS (WHOOPING COUGH)

Before the introduction of diphtheria/tetanus/pertussis vaccination in the United States in the 1940s, there were on average more than 200,000 cases of pertussis annually with more than 4000 deaths per year.[42] Outbreaks have been observed in communities and on college campuses[43–45] (**Table 5**).

The greatest mortality associated with pertussis occurs in young infants, including those too young to be vaccinated. One attempt to protect newborns, “cocooning”, centers on the vaccination of family members and the postpartum vaccination of the infant’s mother. Data on the efficacy of this strategy are inconclusive.[42] Recent studies suggest that newborns may become infected via transmission of pertussis from their (generally vaccinated) siblings: vaccination prevents infection but does not prevent carriage or transmission of the bacteria. Since 2012, the ACIP has recommended vaccination of women during the third trimester of pregnancy to ensure that antibodies to pertussis will cross the placenta and that newborns will have immunity lasting until they can themselves be vaccinated.[46]

Table 3
Meningococcal disease

Peak ages	• Most cases of meningitis occur in preschool children, with another peak in late teens—early twenties[21] • Identified outbreaks generally occur in the college/university setting, or in the military • For 2011 through 2019, all US university-associated outbreaks have been serogroup B[27]
Key findings on presentation	• Begins with nonspecific symptoms: chills, fever, myalgia, nausea, and vomiting • Then classic features of headache, neck stiffness, photophobia, and altered mental status may develop—but less than one-third of patients present this way[24] • Meningococcal infections may also progress from nonspecific symptoms to shock and purpuric rash (ie, to meningococcemia without meningitis)[24] • A nonblanching hemorrhagic rash is pathognomonic of IMD[24] • In infants, IMD may also present with bulging fontanelle, delayed capillary refill, or seizures[28] • Note that infants and young children may maintain normal blood pressure in the presence of shock. A normal blood pressure, in the presence of other symptoms, may not be reassuring[24,29]
Incubation and infection timing	• Incubation period is 1–10 d (generally <4)[21] • Household contacts of cases have rates of disease 500–800 times the rate in the general population[21] • Patients should be considered contagious for 24 h after beginning appropriate antibiotics[21] • Be aware of asymptomatic carriage: meningococcal disease may be transmitted by persons who do not become ill.[25] Persons who have received conjugate vaccinations against serogroups A, C, W, or Y are less likely to have carriage of those strains; recombinant vaccines against serogroup B may not prevent asymptomatic carriage[3]
Differential includes	• For purpura/petechiae: acute leukemia, idiopathic thrombocytopenic purpura, Henoch-Schonlein purpura[28]
Laboratories	• At the emergency department or hospital setting, lumbar puncture is the main test for meningococcal meningitis and blood culture for meningococcemia[21] • Lumbar puncture can be dangerous in the setting of increased intracranial pressure. Note that CT does not indicate increased intracranial pressure • Other tests for meningococcus include PCR or urine antigen detection[21] • Nasopharyngeal swabs or throat swabs are not helpful for diagnosis. A positive swab may indicate colonization, not infection
If you suspect your patient has invasive meningococcal disease	• The patient needs definitive care immediately. Transfer the patient to the local hospital emergency department ASAP, with droplet precautions • Mortality of IMD is greatly reduced when parenteral antibiotics given before arrival at a hospital.[24,30,31] Cefotaxime and ceftriaxone are the recommended empirical treatments in the United States[21]; parenteral penicillin may also be used. If available, antibiotics should be administered without delaying transportation to emergency department[28]

(continued on next page)

Table 3
(continued)

	• Note: patients can transmit meningococci for 24 h after receiving appropriate antibiotics. Maintain droplet precautions for 24 h • Notify the health department after treatment has begun • The emergent treatment of suspected IMD is beyond the scope of this paper. Nadel, 2016[24] may be a useful reference
Care of contacts	• Chemoprophylaxis can include ciprofloxacin (starting at age 1 mo, excluding pregnant patients); rifampin (all ages, but not pregnant); or ceftriaxone (all ages and can be used in pregnancy)[3,32] as an interim measure before vaccination. Close contacts should receive chemoprophylaxis even if immunized[21]
Guidelines for school, day care, college, etc.	• According to the CDC, the definition of an outbreak as a threshold for considering mass vaccination at an organization such as a university depends on the size of organization and the time course of cases. Generally, 2 cases in 3 mo will be "outbreak"—but in a school with more than 20,000 students, it may need 3 cases to constitute an outbreak[33] • The serogroup of the strain involved in outbreak will determine which vaccines may be appropriate
In health care settings	• Droplet precautions are recommended in addition to standard precautions for 24 h after the initiation of appropriate antibiotics[21]

Abbreviations: CDC, Centers for Disease Control and Prevention; CT, computed tomograph.

Table 4
Hepatitis A

Peak ages	• Highest incidence in ages 20–29 y[38] • Lowest in children through age 9 y[38]—but that may be because most children younger than 6 y who develop hepatitis A are asymptomatic[39]
Key findings on presentation	• Jaundice (70%+); nausea, vomiting, and diarrhea; abdominal pain; weight loss • Hepatomegaly or splenomegaly may be present[39] • Key items in history include exposure to raw food, contaminated drinking water, or exposure to fecal contamination
Incubation and infection timing	• Incubation period lasts approximately 28 d (range: 15–50)[39] • The disease is contagious 2 wk before and at least 1 wk after the onset of symptoms[39]
Differential includes[39]	• Other hepatitis viruses • Other viral or bacterial infection (cytomegalovirus, EBV, typhoid, leptospirosis) • Parasites (liver flukes, toxocariasis) • Systemic lupus erythematosus
Laboratories	• Elevated ALT, AST, total and direct bilirubin • Usually diagnosed by HAV IgM[38] • Make get a false-positive IgM if the patient recently received HAV vaccine[39]
If you suspect your patient has hepatitis A	• Notify health department

(*continued on next page*)

Table 4 (*continued*)	
	• Patients should not return to work or school until fever and jaundice subside
Care of contacts	• If at least 12 mo old and not previously vaccinated, can give single dose of single-antigen vaccine.[38] Can also use Ig.[39] Ig may also be used also for immunocompromised patients, those with chronic liver disease, or if vaccine contraindicated[38]
Guidelines for school, day care, college, etc.	• Postexposure prophylaxis should be offered to those in close contact with the patient, as well as staff members and attendees of child care centers
In health care settings	• Observe standard precautions
Community outreach	• Outreach to homeless populations • If limited supply of vaccine is available, consider running titers before vaccinating[40] • Recommendations to fully vaccinate against hepatitis A and hepatitis B require multiple doses of vaccine. A single dose of HAV vaccine can be 95% effective and has been shown to stop outbreaks[41]

Abbreviations: ALT, alanine aminotransferase; AST, aspartate aminotransferase.

Table 5 Pertussis	
Peak ages	• Infants have highest incidence, but adolescents and adults account for more cases[47]
Key findings on presentation	• Disease is marked by 3 stages: catarrhal, paroxysmal, and convalescence • Not generally noted during catarrhal phase, 1–2 wk • Infants can be apneic to start • Then comes paroxysmal phase, marked by whooping and/or posttussive vomiting • In adults the catarrhal phase is marked by low-grade fever, mild cough, and lacrimation • Paroxysmal phase is much less likely to cause whooping in adults, but patients may still have coughing paroxysms, with the cough worse at night • Neither immunization nor infection provide lifelong immunity, so the history of either is not completely reassuring
Incubation and infection timing	• Incubation period 7–10 d[43] • Infected persons are most contagious through the third wk after the beginning of the catarrhal stage[48]
Differential includes	• Viral upper respiratory infection; sinusitis; postinfectious cough; reaction to ACE inhibitors; gastroesophageal reflux[43]
Laboratories	• Nasopharyngeal swab or aspirate from the *posterior* nasopharynx. Anterior nasopharyngeal swabs or throat

(*continued on next page*)

Table 5
(*continued*)

	swabs have an unacceptably high false-negative rate.[49] Can also use PCR • If using serology, IgM and IgA lack specificity. Elevation in IgG after 2 wk of cough suggests pertussis[49]

If you suspect your patient has pertussis	• Notify your health department
	• Treat with azithromycin or erythromycin. Azithromycin is a shorter course, with less gastrointestinal upset in adults and lower risk of hypertrophic pyloric stenosis in neonates
	  ○ Erythromycin: 40–50 mg/kg/d divided q6h for 14 d, up to 2 g/d divided q6h[50]
	  ○ Azithromycin: 10 mg/kg on day 1, then 5 mg/kg for 4 more days, up to 500 mg on first day and 250 mg for the remainder
	  ○ Other treatments include clarithromycin (7 d) or trimethoprim-sulfamethoxazole (TMP-SMZ) (14 d).[47,50] TMP-SMZ should not be used in infants younger than 2 mo[49]
	• Antibiotics shorten the course of the illness, especially when given early; they also minimize spread to others

Care of contacts	• "Administration of postexposure prophylaxis to asymptomatic household contacts within 21 d of onset of cough in index patient can prevent symptomatic infection"[47] • If pertussis strongly suspected, try to get prophylaxis to close contacts without waiting for confirmation. Prophylaxis of pregnant women and infants should not be delayed[49] • Vaccination should be offered to unimmunized or underimmunized contacts,[48] but vaccination is not a substitute for prophylaxis in persons already exposed.[49] Medications for chemoprophylaxis are the same as those used for treatment[48]
Guidelines for school, day care, college, etc	• Children and child care providers who have symptoms or confirmed pertussis should be excluded from day care or school pending the completion of 5 d of recommended antibiotics. Untreated children should be excluded until 21 d after the onset of cough[48]
In health care settings	• Droplet precautions for 21 d after onset of cough or for 5 d from start of effective antibiotics[48] • Health care providers are recommended to have single dose of Tdap in adulthood; no extra vaccination is suggested because of health care status. If exposed, consider postexposure prophylaxis for those in contact with people at risk of severe disease

Abbreviations: ACE, angiotensin converting enzyme; Tdap, tetanus, diphtheria, and pertussis.

SUMMARY

- Vaccine-preventable diseases continue to occur in outbreaks across the United States. Outbreaks are more likely in communities with lower rates of vaccination and links to regions experiencing outbreaks, but no area can be considered free from potential disease.

- Clinicians need to be familiar with the presentation and recommended treatment of vaccine-preventable diseases.
- Measles outbreaks may occur in regions where less than 92% of the population is immune. The disease spreads rapidly. Isolation and vaccination are major factors in controlling outbreaks.
- Mumps outbreaks are often associated with even highly vaccinated college and university populations. Isolation and vaccination are essential.
- Invasive meningococcal disease develops over a matter of hours. If IMD is suspected, the patient needs immediate transfer using droplet precautions to an appropriate health care facility, such as an emergency department. Transportation and diagnostic studies should not delay administration of appropriate parenteral antibiotics.
- Hepatitis A outbreaks may take place over a large geographic area, if the infection is being carried on widely distributed food products. Conversely, they may also be associated with locally limited sanitation, as occurs for those experiencing homelessness.
- Pertussis continues to have its highest mortality rate among those infants too young to receive vaccines. Vaccination during the third trimester of pregnancy reduces the rate of disease among young infants.
- Coordination and consultation with one's local health department is a vital aspect of managing vaccine-preventable illness.

ACKNOWLEDGMENTS

The author would like to thank Dr Paul Hunter for his help in developing the outline and main themes of this article.

DISCLOSURE

The author has nothing to disclose.

REFERENCES

1. Letley L, Rew V, Ahmed R, et al. Tailoring immunisation programmes: Using behavioural insights to identify barriers and enablers to childhood immunisations in a Jewish community in London, UK. Vaccine 2018;36(31):4687–92.
2. Olive JK, Hotez PJ, Damania A, et al. The state of the antivaccine movement in the United States: A focused examination of nonmedical exemptions in states and counties. PLoS Med 2018;15(6):e1002578.
3. McNamara LA, MacNeil JR, Cohn AC, et al. Mass chemoprophylaxis for control of outbreaks of meningococcal disease. Lancet Infect Dis 2018;18(9):e272–81.
4. CDC Press Releases: ACIP votes down use of LAIV for 2016-2017 flu season. CDC. 2016. Available at: http://www.cdc.gov/media/releases/2016/s0622-laiv-flu.html. Accessed August 13, 2016.
5. Gastanaduy PA, Redd SB, Clemmons NS, et al. Measles. In: Centers for Disease Control and Prevention, editor. Manual for the surveillance of vaccine-preventable diseases. Atlanta (GA): Centers for Disease Control and Prevention; 2017. Available at: https://www.cdc.gov/vaccines/pubs/surv-manual/chpt07-measles.pdf.
6. Roush S. Enhancing Surveillance. In: Centers for Disease Control and Prevention, editor. Manual for the surveillance of vaccine-preventable diseases. Atlanta (GA): Centers for Disease Control and Prevention; 2017.
7. Moss WJ. Measles. Lancet 2017;390(10111):2490–502.

8. American Academy of Pediatrics. Summaries of Infectious Diseases: Measles. In: Kimberlin DW, Brady MT, Jackson MA, et al, editors. Red book: 2018 report of the committee on infectious diseases. 31st edition. Itasca (NY): American Academy of Pediatrics; 2018. p. 537–50.
9. Patel M, Lee AD, Redd SB, et al. Increase in Measles Cases — United States, January 1–April 26, 2019. MMWR Morb Mortal Wkly Rep 2019;68:402–4.
10. Strebel PM, Orenstein WA. Measles. N Engl J Med 2019;381(4):349–57.
11. Measles | Specimen Collection, Storage, and Shipment | Lab Tools | CDC. 2019. Available at: https://www.cdc.gov/measles/lab-tools/rt-pcr.html. Accessed September 1, 2019.
12. Cardemil CV, Dahl RM, James L, et al. Effectiveness of a third dose of MMR vaccine for mumps outbreak control. N Engl J Med 2017;377(10):947–56.
13. Albertson JP. Mumps outbreak at a university and recommendation for a third dose of measles-mumps-rubella vaccine — Illinois, 2015–2016. MMWR Morb Mortal Wkly Rep 2016;65:731–4.
14. Clemmons NS, Hickman CJ, Lee AD, et al. Mumps. In: Centers for Disease Control and Prevention, editor. Manual for the prevention of vaccine-preventable diseases. Atlanta (GA): Centers for Disease Control and Prevention; 2017. Available at: https://www.cdc.gov/vaccines/pubs/surv-manual/chpt09-mumps.pdf.
15. Zamir CS, Schroeder H, Shoob H, et al. Characteristics of a large mumps outbreak: Clinical severity, complications and association with vaccination status of mumps outbreak cases. Hum Vaccines Immunother 2015;11(6):1413–7.
16. Marx GE, Burakoff A, Barnes M, et al. Mumps Outbreak in a Marshallese Community — Denver Metropolitan Area, Colorado, 2016–2017. Morb Mortal Wkly Rep 2018;67(41):1143–6.
17. Tiffany A, Shannon D, Mamtchueng W, et al. Notes from the field: Mumps outbreak — Alaska, May 2017–July 2018. Morb Mortal Wkly Rep 2018;67(33):940–1.
18. Magurano F, Baggieri M, Marchi A, et al. Mumps clinical diagnostic uncertainty. Eur J Public Health 2018;28(1):119–23.
19. Marin M, Marlow M, Moore KL, et al. Recommendation of the Advisory Committee on Immunization Practices for use of a third dose of mumps virus-containing vaccine in persons at increased risk for mumps during an outbreak. MMWR Morb Mortal Wkly Rep 2018;67(1):33–8.
20. American Academy of Pediatrics. Summaries of Infectious Diseases: Mumps. In: Kimberlin DW, Brady MT, Jackson MA, et al, editors. Red book: 2018 report of the committee on infectious diseases. 31st edition. Itasca (NY): American Academy of Pediatrics; 2018. p. 567–73.
21. American Academy of Pediatrics. Summaries of Infectious Diseases: Meningococcal Infections. In: Kimberlin DW, Brady MT, Jackson MA, et al, editors. Red book: 2018 report of the committee on infectious diseases. 31st edition. Itasca (NY): American Academy of Pediatrics; 2018. p. 551–61.
22. Manage meningococcal disease risk in patients taking eculizumab | CDC. 2019. Available at: https://www.cdc.gov/meningococcal/clinical/eculizumab.html. Accessed September 23, 2019.
23. Harrison LH, Shutt KA, Arnold KE, et al. Meningococcal carriage among Georgia and Maryland high school students. J Infect Dis 2015;211(11):1761–8.
24. Nadel S. Treatment of meningococcal disease. J Adolesc Health 2016;59(2, Supplement):S21–8.

25. CDC Press Releases: Meningococcal Disease Update. CDC. 2016. Available at: https://www.cdc.gov/media/releases/2014/s0318-meningococcal-diisease.html. Accessed September 16, 2019.
26. Meningococcal - Information, Communicable Disease Service. Available at: https://www.nj.gov/health/cd/meningo/update2013-2014.shtml. Accessed September 23, 2019.
27. Soeters HM, McNamara LA, Blain AE, et al. University-based outbreaks of meningococcal disease caused by serogroup B, United States, 2013–2018. Emerg Infect Dis 2019;25(3):434–40.
28. Thomas AE, Baird SF, Anderson J. Purpuric and petechial rashes in adults and children: initial assessment. BMJ 2016;352:i1285.
29. Hamilton JL, John SP. Evaluation of fever in infants and young children. Am Fam Physician 2013;87(4):254–60.
30. Cartwright K, Strang J, Gossain S, et al. Early treatment of meningococcal disease. BMJ 1992;305(6856):774.
31. Strang JR, Pugh EJ. Meningococcal infections: Reducing the case fatality rate by giving penicillin before admission to hospital. BMJ 1992;305(6846):141–3.
32. Antibiotics for preventing meningococcal infections - Zalmanovici Trestioreanu, A - 2013 | Cochrane Library. Available at: https://www-cochranelibrary-com/cdsr/doi/10.1002/14651858.CD004785.pub5/full. Accessed September 2, 2019.
33. Centers for Disease Control and Prevention. Guidance for the evaluation and public health management of suspected outbreaks of meningococcal disease. 2017. Available at: https://www.cdc.gov/meningococcal/downloads/meningococcal-outbreak-guidance.pdf. Accessed September 8, 2019.
34. Gossner CM, Severi E. Three simultaneous, food-borne, multi-country outbreaks of hepatitis A virus infection reported in EPIS-FWD in 2013: what does it mean for the European Union? Euro Surveill 2014;19(43):20941.
35. Hosseini M, Ding A. Hepatitis A outbreak in San Diego county, 2016–2017: A morphologic and epidemiologic review. Open Forum Infect Dis 2018;5(Suppl 1):S646.
36. How the City is addressing Philadelphia's hepatitis A outbreak | Department of Public Health. City of Philadelphia. Available at: https://www.phila.gov/2019-08-30-how-the-city-is-addressing-philadelphias-hepatitis-a-outbreak/. Accessed September 23, 2019.
37. Doshani M, Weng M, Moore KL, et al. Recommendations of the Advisory Committee on Immunization Practices for use of Hepatitis A vaccine for persons experiencing homelessness. Morb Mortal Wkly Rep 2019;68(6):153–6.
38. Hofmeister MG, Klevens M, Nelson NP. Hepatitis A. In: Centers for Disease Control and Prevention, editor. Manual for the surveillance of vaccine-preventable diseases. Atlanta (GA): 2017. Available at: https://www.cdc.gov/vaccines/pubs/surv-manual/chpt03-hepa.html. Accessed September 2, 2019.
39. Matheny SC, Kingery JE. Hepatitis A. Am Fam Physician 2012;86(11):1027–34.
40. Campos-Outcalt D. CDC provides advice on recent hepatitis A outbreaks. J Fam Pract 2018;67:30.
41. Outbreak-specific considerations for hepatitis A vaccine administration | CDC. 2019. Available at: https://www.cdc.gov/hepatitis/outbreaks/InterimOutbreakGuidance-HAV-VaccineAdmin.htm. Accessed September 8, 2019.
42. Liang JL, Tiwari T, Moro P, et al. Recommendations and reports: Prevention of pertussis, tetanus, and diphtheria with vaccines in the United States: Recommendations of the Advisory Committee on Immunization Practices (ACIP). MMWR Recomm Rep 2018;67(2):1–42.

43. Spector TB, Maziarz EK. Pertussis. Med Clin North Am 2013;97(4):537–52.
44. Matthias J, Dusek C, Pritchard PS, et al. Outbreak of pertussis in a school and religious community averse to health care and vaccinations — Columbia County, Florida, 2013. MMWR Morb Mortal Wkly Rep 2014;63(30):655.
45. Local health department costs associated with response to a school-based pertussis outbreak — Omaha, Nebraska, September–November 2008. MMWR Morb Mortal Wkly Rep 2011;60(1):5–9.
46. Centers for Disease Control and Prevention (CDC). Updated recommendations for use of tetanus toxoid, reduced diphtheria toxoid, and acellular pertussis vaccine (Tdap) in pregnant women–Advisory Committee on Immunization Practices (ACIP), 2012. MMWR Morb Mortal Wkly Rep 2013;62(7):131–5.
47. Recommended antimicrobial agents for the treatment and postexposure prophylaxis of pertussis: 2005 CDC guidelines. Available at: https://www.cdc.gov/mmwr/preview/mmwrhtml/rr5414a1.htm. Accessed September 8, 2019.
48. American Academy of Pediatrics. Summaries of infectious diseases: Pertussis (Whooping Cough). In: Kimberlin DW, Brady MT, Jackson MA, et al, editors. Red book: 2018 report of the committee on infectious diseases. 31st edition. Itasca (NY): American Academy of Pediatrics; 2018. p. 620–34.
49. Faulkner A, Skoff T, Cassiday P, et al. Pertussis. In: Manual for the surveillance of vaccine-preventable diseases. Atlanta (GA): Centers for Disease Control and Prevention; 2017. Available at: http://www.cdc.gov/pertussis/surv-reporting.html. Accessed November 17, 2014.
50. Cherry JD. Treatment of pertussis—2017. J Pediatr Infect Dis Soc 2018;7(3):e123–5.

Addressing Immunization Health Disparities

Melissa L. Martinez, MD[a,*], Sarah Coles, MD[b]

KEYWORDS

• Vaccine • Disparity • Immunization

KEY POINTS

- Vaccine disparities based on many factors, such as race and ethnicity, economic status, and rural versus urban locations of residents, are ongoing issues in the United States.
- Reasons for disparities include cost, access, coverage, attitudes/beliefs, and systems issues.
- Systems, such as the Vaccines for Children program, revisions to Medicaid, and funding provided under section 371 of the Vaccine Assistance Act, in some cases, narrowed disparities but gaps continue.
- At a practice level, several measures can help ensure that every patient is offered recommended vaccines and address disparities.

Three million lives are saved each year by vaccines throughout the world.[1] Unfortunately, in the United States, vaccination rates differ between racial/ethnic groups, geographic areas of residence, income levels, disabilities, and other factors. This article reviews some of the disparities in vaccination in the United States and offers approaches to address disparities to realize the full benefit of vaccines for all people.

DISPARITIES

Race and Ethnicity

Limitations of data on race and ethnicity

Coverage rate data for race/ethnicity come with some significant limitations. The main source of data is the Centers for Disease Control and Prevention and other governmental surveys. In some cases, survey data are confirmed by a review of provider records, but the data mostly are reliant on reports of responders.[2,3] Definitions and reporting of race/ethnicity differ between studies, often grouping racial and ethnic minorities into a single catch-all category. For example, American Indians and Alaska

[a] Department of Internal Medicine, University of New Mexico, Health Sciences Center, 801 Encino Place Northeast, C14, Albuquerque, NM 87102, USA; [b] Department of Family, Community and Preventive Medicine, Family Medicine Residency, University of Arizona College of Medicine - Phoenix, 1300 North 12th Street #605, Phoenix, AZ 85006, USA
* Corresponding author.
E-mail address: MLMartinez@salud.unm.edu

Prim Care Clin Office Pract 47 (2020) 483–495
https://doi.org/10.1016/j.pop.2020.05.004
0095-4543/20/

Natives (AI/AN) as well as those who report belonging to more than 1 racial group are classified in a single category, called "other."[4]

Race and ethnicity are not mutually exclusive. For example, Hispanic individuals may identify as any race. Coverage rates by race are not homogeneous. In a survey conducted in California, Asians seemed to have higher likelihood of receiving influenza vaccine than whites, but on subgroup analysis, only Koreans and Vietnamese had higher vaccination rates.[5] This diversity of rates likely is true for other racial and ethnic groupings. Despite these challenges, available data show a pattern of difference in vaccination rates by race and ethnicity, with greater differences for adults than for children or adolescents.

Racial/ethnic rates in children

There are higher rates for vaccines in children than in adults, and children are less likely to have statistically lower disparity between racial/ethnic groups (**Fig. 1**).[4,6,7] For example, in children, ages 19 months to 35 months, completion of the combined 7-vaccine series for non-Hispanic black and AI/AN children are not statistically lower than for non-Hispanic white and Asian children (**Fig. 2**).[8] The wide confidence levels overlap due to low response rates in these groups. Data from 2006 to 2010 demonstrated no difference in vaccination rates found for AI/AN children compared with those of other races.[9,10] The Indian Health Service reports comparable rates for age-appropriate vaccination for children 3 months to 27 months of age in the second quarter of 2019. These data are reported for AI/AN children seen within the Indian Health Service system and do not necessarily reflect the rates for this racial group as a whole.

Racial/ethnic rates in adolescents

Rates of Tdap (tetanus, diphtheria and acellular pertussis vaccine) for adolescents were not substantially different for most races/ethnicities except for Hispanics, who had a slightly lower rate.[11] Rate of conjugate meningitis vaccine were higher for blacks, Hispanics, and Asians than for white non-Hispanics.[11] Rates for AI/AN were comparable to those of whites. There were no differences in the rates of measles,

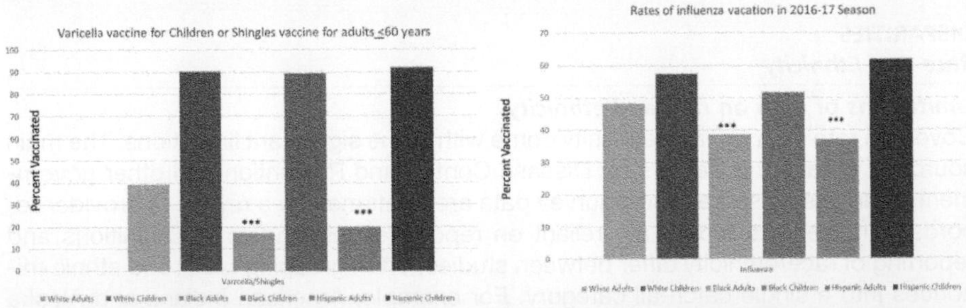

Fig. 1. Rates Adults and Children in Selected Vaccines 2017. Although, vaccines in adults and children are not strictly comparable, this graph is intended to demonstrate differences in disparities in adults versus children. Over all children have higher rates of recommended vaccines and smaller differences between Non-Hispanic whites versus Non-Hispanic blacks and Hispanics. In fact only in adults are differences between Non-Hispanic Whites and other groups statistically significant. ***Statistically significant difference between White versus Black or Hispanic Adults. (*Data from* Centers for Disease Control and Prevention. Vaccination coverage among adults in the United States, National Health Interview Survey, 2017. Available at: https://www.cdc.gov/vaccines/imz-managers/coverage/adultvaxview/pubs-resources/NHIS-2017.htm; and Centers for Disease Control and Prevention. National Immunization Survey Children 2017 supplemental table. Available at: https://stacks.cdc.gov/view/cdc/59414.)

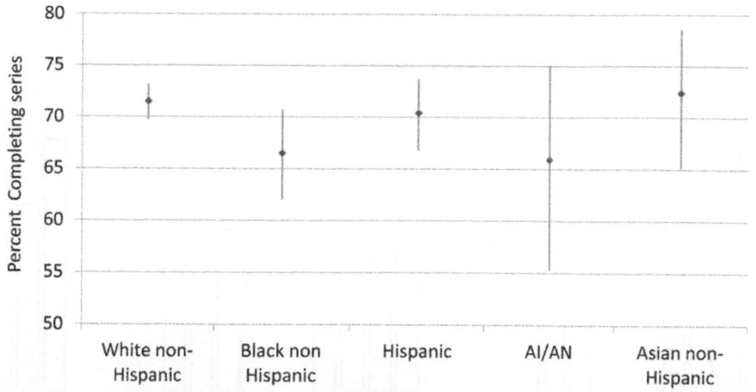

Fig. 2. Rate of 7 Vaccine Series in Children 19-35 Months in 2017. (*Data from* Centers for Disease Control and Prevention. National Immunization Survey Children 2017 supplemental table. Available at: https://stacks.cdc.gov/view/cdc/59414.)

measles, mumps. rubella vaccine (MMR); hepatitis B vaccine; or varicella vaccine but ANs/NIs had a much higher rate of immunity acquired by having the disease.[12]

Racial/ethnic disparity in adults

Asian adults have the highest rate of influenza vaccination followed by white, black, Hispanic, and AN/AI adults[13] (**Fig. 3**). White adults have higher rates of tetanus and pertussis vaccines[14] (**Fig. 4**). White adults ages 65 and up are more likely to have received pneumococcal, live shingles, and tetanus vaccines than other groups (**Fig. 5**).[15] A review of claims data filed for those greater or equal to 65 years old, indicated that 45.6% of white non-Hispanics, 36.3% of black non-Hispanics, 30% of

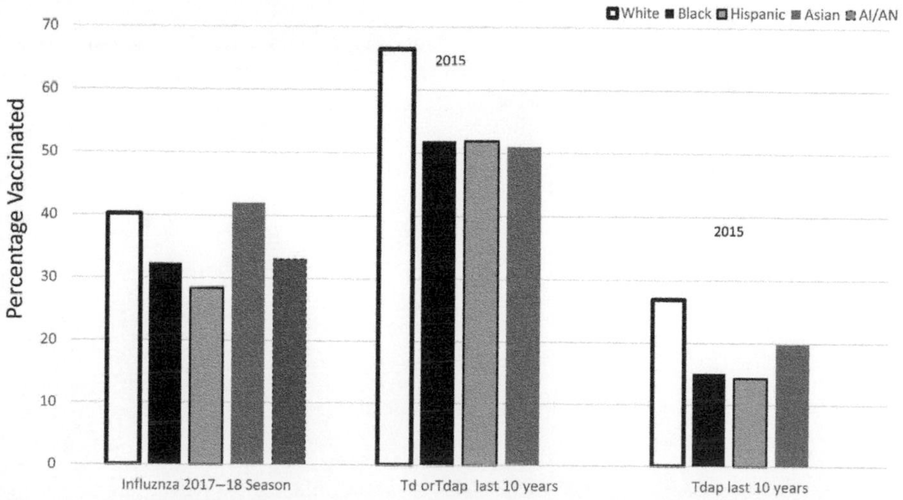

Fig. 3. Percentage of adults age greater than age 18 who received selected vaccines. (*Data from* Centers for Disease Control and Prevention. 2016-2017 flu season data. Available at: https://www.cdc.gov/flu/fluvaxview/coverage-1617estimates.htm; and Williams WW, Lu P-J, O'Halloran A, et al. Surveillance of vaccination coverage among adult populations — United States, 2015. MMWR Surveill Summ. 2017;66(11):1-28.)

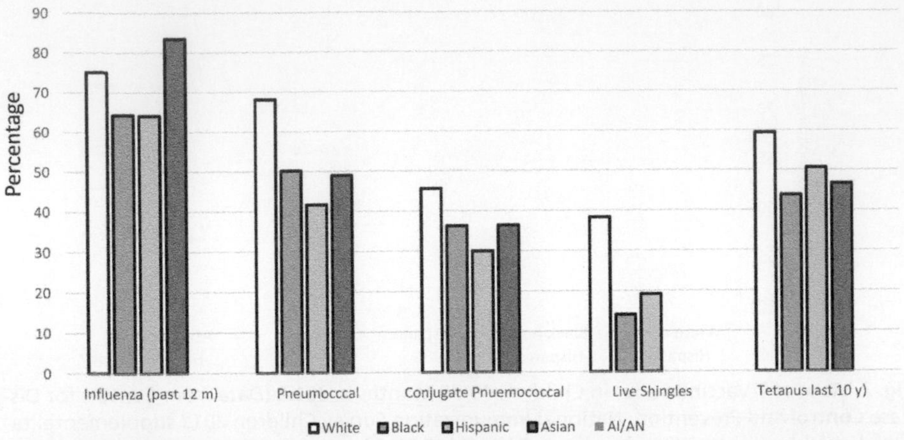

Fig. 4. Percentage of adults ages greater than or equal to 65 years who received selected vaccines. (*Data from* Norris T, Vahratian A, Cohen RA. Vaccination coverage among adults aged 65 and over: United States, 2015. NCHS Data Brief. 2017;(281):1-8; and McLaughlin JM, Swerdlow DL, Khan F, et al. Disparities in uptake of 13-valent pneumococcal conjugate vaccine among older adults in the United States. Hum Vaccines Immunother. 2019;15(4):841-849.)

Hispanics, and 44.2% of Asians had received pneumococcal conjugate vaccine (PCV13) in 2017.[16]

Influenza and pertussis (Tdap) vaccines are important, especially in pregnancy. In an Internet panel survey of pregnant women, white women had a higher rate of Tdap and influenza vaccine than black non-Hispanic, Hispanic, or women of other races (59.3%, 42.9%, 48.8%, and 56.5% respectively).[17]

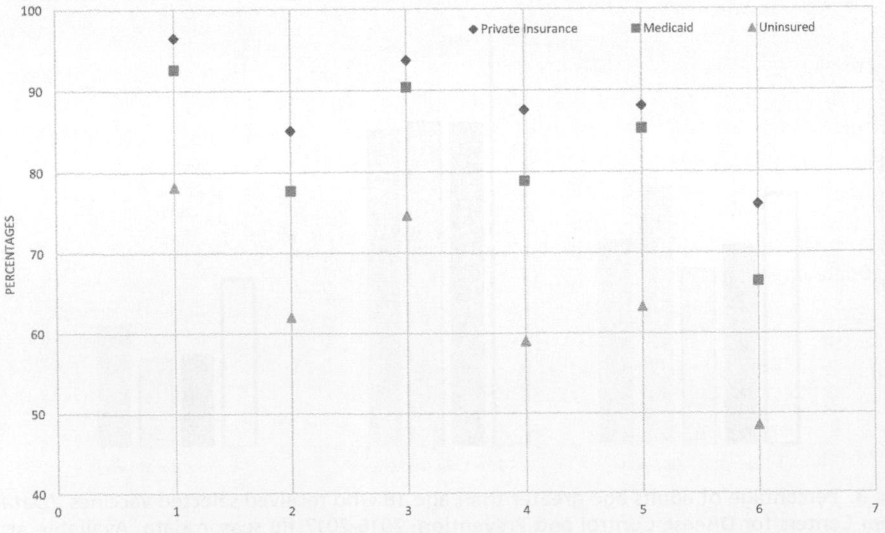

1: DTaP ≥3 doses; 2: Hib, full; 3: MMR ≥1 dose; 4: PCV ≥4 doses; 5: HepA(Hepatitis A Vaccine) ≥1 dose; 6: Combined 7 Vaccine Series

Fig. 5. Vaccination rates by health insurance status, children ages 19 months to 35 months.

Income and Poverty

Adults and children living at or below 100% of the poverty level routinely have lower vaccination rates than individuals living above the poverty level.[6,8] For human papillomavirus vaccine (HPV), adolescents living below the poverty level had higher rates of HPV completion (53.7%) than those living above the poverty level (46.7%).[11]

Adults living at or below 100% of the poverty level have lower rates of influenza and pneumococcal vacations compared with higher-income groups.[18,19] There is a correlation with higher income and higher rates of influenza and pertussis vaccine in pregnant women.[5]

The inactivated shingles vaccine, recommended for all persons age greater than or equal to 60, is an extreme example of disparity base on income.[20] This vaccine was covered only as the Medicare Part D (pharmacy) benefit. Persons who were poor had less than half the rate of shingles vaccination (14.8%) than those who were not poor (39.6%).[15]

Insurance

In 2018%, 9.4% (30.4 million) of people in the United States had no insurance coverage: 5.2% of American children and 13.3% of adults.[21] Vaccination rates are lower for most vaccines in children ages 19 months to 35 months who are covered by Medicaid or uninsured compared with private health insurance (see **Fig. 5**).[8] This difference exists despite the Vaccines for Children (VFC) program, which provides free vaccines to uninsured children and children with Medicaid.[9] The disparity is most evident in for the diphtheria, tetanus, and pertussis vaccine (DTaP); *Haemophilus influenzae* type B vaccine (Hib); and PCV series—vaccines that require a booster dosing during second year of life.[9] In 2015%, 17.2% of uninsured children received no vaccines compared with 0.8% of children with private insurance.[8] Less than half of uninsured children received all recommended vaccines in the combined 7-vaccine series. Similarly, vaccination coverage is significantly lower among uninsured adolescents compared with insured adolescents for vaccines and doses except for completions of HPV vaccines in males.[11,22] For insured adults, individuals with private insurance have higher rates than those reporting public health insurance.[14]

Geographic

Rates of vacations are reported for areas of residence in metropolitan statistical areas (MSAs): MSA principal city, MSA nonprincipal city, and non-MSA. MSAs contain at least 1 urbanized area of 50,000 people or more.[11,14]

Vaccination rates for children and adults living outside of MSAs are lower than those living in cities.[23] The rural versus urban difference is most pronounced in the rates of HPV for adolescents.[24] Vanderpool and colleagues[25] noted an "incongruence of low HPV vaccination coverage in geographic regions with high HPV-associated disease..." For adults, pneumococcal rates are only slightly lower for persons with a residence outside an MSA compared with those in an MSA.[18] The rate of PCV13 in persons ages 65 and older in rural areas was 22.9% compared with 45.8% in suburban area and 33.8% in urban areas.[16]

FACTORS CONTRIBUTING TO DISPARITIES

The Role of Bias

The word, *bias*, has emotional connotations, but bias can be unconscious, unintended, and institutional. The role that institutional bias has in disparities is hard to recognize and measure. Approximately one-third of African Americans, in 1 study, stated they have personally experienced racial discrimination in health care and 22% have avoided seeking medical care out of concern for discrimination.[26] Implicit bias is significantly related to differences in patient-physician interactions, treatment decisions, treatment adherence, and patient health outcomes.[27]

In a 2011 to 2012 survey of patients with chronic conditions, 7.3% reported experiencing a time when they perceived discrimination in a health care setting, and these patients had lower rates of influenza vaccination compared with those with no reported discrimination.[28] Theoretically, all eligible veterans attending Veterans Administration hospitals should have equal access to influenza vaccines. But in 2006, white Veterans Administration patients had an influenza vaccination rate of 82%, higher than that of blacks (71%), Hispanics (79%), and AIs/ANs (74%).[29]

Acceptance

The 2019 outbreaks of measles highlight the impact that social, cultural, and familial beliefs and attitudes can have vaccine uptake. A majority of outbreaks occurred in close-knit communities with low rates of vaccine coverage[30,31] A similar pattern has been noticed in other communities, where there is greater but not universal rejection of vaccine recommendations.[32,33] Social and community norms, media, misinformation, distrust of systems, and individual experiences can influence vaccine acceptance.[34,35]

Quinn[36] found that black non-Hispanic adults have lower knowledge and trust in influenza vaccines and perceived more barriers to getting vaccines than white non-Hispanics. Lack of trust in the health care system due to a history of discrimination in minority populations can have a negative impact on acceptance of vaccines.[37,38]

Access to Immunizations

Access and convenience are key factors in predicting the likelihood of getting vaccinated.[22,37,39–41]

Access to Health Care Providers

A health care provider recommendation is critical to patients accepting and receiving vaccines.[41–46] Individuals with recent medical visits and/or a usual place for health care report higher vaccination rates, regardless of health insurance status.[11,14,19,22,41,43]

Rural areas have fewer physicians and primary care clinics. Those who live in these areas also face social, logistical, and financial barriers in accessing available health care.[45] Predominately white service areas had more health care services compared with predominantly minority service areas.[46]

Affordability

Cost concerns have an impact on both patients and clinicians.[37,47] Concerns about cost often are cited as one reason not to get vaccinated[39,40] Vaccine costs can be a barrier if patients or health care providers perceive that the vaccine is not covered or expensive.[47] The only vaccines covered by Medicare Part B are influenza, pneumococcal, tetanus, and hepatitis B.[48,49] Medicare Part D covers other recommended vaccines but often with copays. In a Government Accountability Office survey conducted in 2010, physicians reported that Medicare patients declined Part D covered vaccines more frequently than Part B covered vaccines due to concerns about costs and lack of part D coverage.[48]

Although the Affordable Care Act (ACA) helped improve coverage, it did not eliminate financial barriers for patients or providers. States can opt to expand Medicaid, although not every state elected to do so. Each state determines covered vaccines in Medicaid program, cost-sharing, provider reimbursement, and the settings where vaccines are covered.[49,50] States where Medicaid covered influenza vaccines saw a significantly higher rate of influenza vaccination than states without coverage.[51,52]

SYSTEMS-BASED SOLUTIONS

Vaccines for Children

Children who are insured by Medicaid, uninsured, or AIs/ANs are eligible for the VFC program. Approximately 50% of children under the age of 19 are eligible for the VFC program.[9] This program is responsible for the overall high rates of vaccination in US children and has been credited with reducing, although not eliminating, racial and income disparities[9,10]

VFC helped to transition immunization delivery in public health clinics to private practices and helped to provide this crucial care in the patient's medical home. Analysis from 2009 demonstrated that for each dollar invested in vaccination, $3 in direct benefits and $10 in indirect benefits were obtained.[53]

Cost to Practices and Patients

The Community Preventive Services Task Force recommend reducing out-of-pocket costs as a means of increasing rates of vaccine in children, adolescents, and adults.[54] Costs to purchase, store, and administer vaccines, including management of vaccination programs and billing, impair practice participation in vaccination.[49,55] Most physicians do not stock the shingles vaccine due to the cost of purchasing a supply and Part D billing challenges.[49,56]

Although the ACA helped improve coverage, especially for adults, it did not eliminate financial barriers for physicians. Under the ACA, recommended vaccines must be given without copays but the rate of provider reimbursement is not specified.[49] Medicaid coverage also varies by state,[49] further complicating administrative and knowledge barriers for physicians. Many providers indicated dissatisfaction with Medicare and Medicaid and a lack of understanding of covered vaccines under the ACA.[47] Unifying state Medicaid coverage of vaccines and minimizing out-of-pocket costs for Medicaid enrollees can reduce disparities.

ADDRESSING VACCINE DISPARITIES IN PRIMARY CARE PRACTICES

No single intervention to decrease vaccine disparity works for every practice. Each practice should utilize a targeted intervention for its practice style, community, and identified needs. Ideas to assist practices in addressing vaccine disparities are discussed.

Analyze the Demographics and Vaccinations Rates in the Practice Population

The practice identifies a target population (for example, the population in the community or the population of patients in the practice). Looking at the rates for all vaccines may be overwhelming. Focusing on a specific vaccine and populations can limit the project to manageable data set. Not all practices have easy access to useful data[57];

participation in state-run immunization information systems registries may enable practices to generate practice-level reports on immunization rates.[58] Tracking rates of immunization over time allows practices to see trends, develop strategies to address disparities, and monitor the success of interventions.

Analyze Barriers to Immunizations in Disproportionally Affected Populations

Barriers might include cultural divides, transportation, and financial issues.[57,59] Patients and/or community leaders are excellent resources to find out why patients in a specific community are not getting vaccines.[37] Practice staff who live in the community may provide helpful insight. Practices can identify, partner with, and refer to community resources to address unmet needs.

Standardize Practice Procedures that Promote Vaccinations

A recent review cites "a lack of systems that hardwire vaccination into clinical practice" as a cause of disparity.[37] A regular source of health care and a systematic approach by clinics can reduce disparities.[60]

One model is the 4 Pillars Program, a Web-based tool kit for practices.[61] The 4 Pillars Program includes convenient vaccination services, patient communication, enhanced office systems to facilitate immunization, and office champions.

Utilization of standing orders and engaging the entire health care team can assist in reducing missed opportunities. Consistent use of statewide immunization information systems can identify patient needs. Other procedures shown to be effective include reminder/recall systems, standing orders, assessment and feedback to providers, open access scheduling, and clinic appointment times available to meet the needs of that population (such as nighttime and weekend hours).[57,58,60,62,63]

Practices should engage stakeholders in the design and implementation of new systems or processes. These could include patients via a patient advisory group or surveys.[37,60]

Develop Strong Messaging

Strong recommendations and offers to administer the vaccine by clinicians greatly increase the likelihood an individual accepts vaccination. Studies show that minority patients do not receive as many vaccine recommendations as non-minority patients.[62,63]

Practices should incorporate immunization recommendations into every clinical encounter to avoid missed oppertunties.[62] Missed opportunities account for 41.6% of children without a measles vaccine.[64] It is estimated that 90% coverage for DTaP, PCV, and Hib for children ages 19 months to 35 months is attainable if missed opportunities for vaccination are eliminated.[53] Strategies to reduce missed opportunities include a clinician practice of "every person, every time."[65,66] Each individual presenting for any care, including acute, chronic, and preventive visits, should be assessed for and offered missing vaccines.

Addressing vaccine refusal and hesitancy is beyond the scope of this article. Utilizing a patient-centered approach, however, that builds trust is recommended.[64] Patient-centered medical care in which the clinician gives adequate time, listens, and is respectful to concerns correlates with higher rates of vaccination.

Tailored messages that are culturally appropriate can improve vaccination acceptance. When designing campaigns to improve acceptance, including representatives from the target population can help create culturally appropriate messaging. Patient educations materials, such as posters or brochures, should offer pictures depicting persons with the race, age, and gender of target populations, be at an appropriate reading level, and be translated into appropriate languages.[36,41] Health literacy is a barrier and clinicians should avoid jargon, work to improve communication skills, and use translation services.[37]

Engage in Community Outreach

Offering vaccines in settings beyond the clinic can increase access. Pharmacies and schools are the sites recommended most often. Physicians can participate in community-based education programs or campaigns.[37] Community organizations, faith communities, civic groups, and other organizations are potential partners for outreach or education.[36,57]

Optimize Immunization Financing

As the models of payment for care shift from fee-for-service to value-based care, vaccinations may become more financially viable for practices.[67] Given the complexity of vaccination reimbursement, many practices likely would benefit from "education and technical assistance related to vaccine financing and billing and greater use of purchasing strategies to decrease upfront vaccine cost."[49,59,67]

Assist with Financial Barrier that Patients Encounter

Practices can participate in programs to help low-income patients access health care resources, such as Medicare, Medicaid, and VFC.

Share Best Practices

Clinicians can work with their community to share ideas and develop best practices. Small pilot projects can be expanded if successful.[57]

SUMMARY

According to the World Health Organization, "Vaccination greatly reduces disease, disability, death and inequity…".[1] The effectiveness of vaccines depends on their ability to reach a majority of eligible people. Primary care practices are crucial in the delivery of vaccines and can help contribute to vaccine equity.

DISCLOSURE

The authors have nothing to disclose.

REFERENCES

1. WHO Value of vaccines. Available at: https://www.who.int/bulletin/volumes/86/2/07-040089/en/. Last Accessed September 29, 2019.
2. National Health Inventory Survey. Available at: https://www.cdc.gov/nchs/nhis/about_nhis.htm. Last Accessed September 29, 2019.
3. National Immunizations Survey. Available at: https://www.cdc.gov/vaccines/imz-managers/nis/index.html. Last Accessed September 22, 2019.
4. Vaccination Coverage among Adults in the United States, National Health Interview Survey. 2017. Available at: https://www.cdc.gov/vaccines/imz-managers/coverage/adultvaxview/pubs-resources/NHIS-2017.htm. Last Accessed June 23 ,2020.
5. Almario CV, May FP, Maxwell AE, et al. Persistent racial and ethnic disparities in flu vaccination coverage: Results from a population-based study. Am J Infect Control 2016;44(9):1004–9.

6. National Immunization Survey Children 2017 Supplemental Table. Available at: https://stacks.cdc.gov/view/cdc/59414. Last Accessed June 23 ,2020.
7. Estimated vaccination coverage among children aged 19 – 35 months, by selected vaccines and doses, race/ethnicity ,* and poverty level † — National Immunization. 2017:2017. Available at: https://stacks.cdc.gov/view/cdc/59415. Last Accessed September 22, 2019.
8. Hill HA, Elam-evans LD, Yankey D, et al. Vaccination coverage among children aged 19 – 35 months — United States, 2015. MMWR Morb Mortal Wkly Rep 2016;65(39):1065–71.
9. Whitney CG, Zhou F, James S, et al. Benefits from immunization during the vaccines for children program era — United States, 1994–2013. Morb Mortal Wkly Rep 2014;63(16):352–5.
10. Walker AT, Smith PJ, Kolasa M. Centers for Disease Control and Prevention (CDC). Reduction of racial/ethnic disparities in vaccination coverage, 1995-2011. MMWR Suppl 2014;63(1):7–12.
11. Walker TY, Elam-Evans LD, Yankey D, et al. National, regional, state, and selected local area vaccination coverage among adolescents aged 13–17 Years — United States, 2017. MMWR Morb Mortal Wkly Rep 2018;67(33):909–17.
12. Indian Health Service. Table FY19 1st and 2nd Quarter Twenty-four to Twenty-seven Month Vaccination Coverage by HIS Areas for FY 2019, Q2. 2019. Available at: https://www.ihs.gov/epi/vaccine/reports/. Last Accessed June 23 ,2020.
13. 2016-2017 Flu Season Data. Available at: https://www.cdc.gov/flu/fluvaxview/coverage-1617estimates.htm. Last Accessed June 22 ,2020.
14. Williams WW, Lu P-J, O'Halloran A, et al. Surveillance of vaccination coverage among adult populations — United States, 2015. MMWR Surveill Summ 2017; 66(11):1–28.
15. Norris T, Vahratian A, Cohen RA. Vaccination Coverage Among Adults Aged 65 and Over: United States, 2015. NCHS Data Brief 2017;281:1–8.
16. McLaughlin JM, Swerdlow DL, Khan F, et al. Disparities in uptake of 13-valent pneumococcal conjugate vaccine among older adults in the United States. Hum Vaccin Immunother 2019;15(4):841–9.
17. Kahn KE, Black CL, Ding H, et al. Influenza and Tdap Vaccination Coverage Among Pregnant Women — United States, April 2018. MMWR Morb Mortal Wkly Rep 2018;67(38):1055–9.
18. Center for Health Statistics N. Table 69. Pneumococcal Vaccination among Adults Aged 18 and over, by Selected Characteristics: United States, Selected Years 1989–2016. 2017. Available at: https://www.cdc.gov/nchs/hus/contents2017.htm#069. Last Accessed June 22, 2020.
19. Center for Health Statistics N. Table 68. Influenza Vaccination among Adults Aged 18 and over, by Selected Characteristics: United States, Selected Years 1989–2016. 2017. Available at: https://www.cdc.gov/nchs/hus/contents2017.htm#068. Last Accessed June 23, 2020.
20. Harpaz R, Ortega-Sanchez IR, Seward M JF. Prevention of Herpes Zoster Recommendations of the Advisory Committee on Immunization Practices (ACIP). MMWR Morb Mortal Wkly Rep 2008;57(05):1–3. Available at: https://www.cdc.gov/mmwr/preview/mmwrhtml/rr5705a1.htm. Last Accessed June 23, 2020.
21. Cohen RA, Terlizzi EP, Martinez ME. P a g e | 1 Health Insurance Coverage: Early Release of Estimates From the National Health Interview Survey, 2018 What's New?. Available at: https://www.cdc.gov/nchs/data/nhis/earlyrelease/insur201905.pdf.

22. Lu PJ, Yankey D, Jeyarajah J, et al. Association of health insurance status and vaccination coverage among adolescents 13-17 years of age. J Pediatr 2018; 195:256–62.e1.
23. Center for Health Statistics N. Table 66. Vaccination Coverage for Selected Diseases among Children Aged 19–35 Months, by Race, Hispanic Origin, Poverty Level, and Location of Residence in Metropolitan Statistical Area: United States, Selected Years 1998–2016. 2017. Available at: https://www.cdc.gov/nchs/hus/contents2017.htm#066. Last Accessed June 23, 2020.
24. National Immunization Survey–Teen (NIS-Teen), United States, 2018. Available at: https://www.cdc.gov/mmwr/volumes/68/wr/mm6833a2.htm#T2_down. Last Accessed June 23, 2020.
25. Vanderpool RC, Stradtman LR, Brandt HM. Policy opportunities to increase HPV vaccination in rural communities. Hum Vaccin Immunother 2018;15(7–8): 1527–32.
26. Discrimination in America: experiences and views of Afircan Americans. NPR and Robert Wood Johnson Foundation; 2018. Available at: https://legacy.npr.org/assets/img/2017/10/23/discriminationpoll-african-americans.pdf. Last Accessed June 23, 2020.
27. Hall WJ, Chapman MV, Lee KM, et al. Implicit racial/ethnic bias among health care professionals and its influence on health care outcomes: A systematic review. Am J Public Health 2015;105(12):e60–76.
28. Bleser WK, Miranda PY, Jean-Jacques M. Racial/ethnic disparities in influenza vaccination of chronically ill US adults the mediating role of perceived discrimination in health care. Med Care 2016;54:570–7.
29. Straits-Tröster KA, Kahwati LC, Kinsinger LS, et al. Racial/ethnic differences in influenza vaccination in the veterans affairs healthcare system. Am J Prev Med 2006;31(5):375–82.
30. Patel M, Lee AD, Redd SB, et al. Increase in Measles Cases - United States, January 1-April 26, 2019. MMWR Morb Mortal Wkly Rep 2019;68(17):402–4.
31. McDonald R, Schnabel Ruppert, et al. Measles Outbreaks from Imported Cases in Orthodox Jewish Communities — New York and New Jersey, 2018–2019. MMWR 2019;68:19.
32. Wooten KG, Wortley PM, Singleton JA, et al. Perceptions matter: Beliefs about influenza vaccine and vaccination behavior among elderly white, black and Hispanic Americans. Vaccine 2012;30(48):6927–34.
33. Wenger OK, McManus MD, Bower JR, et al. Underimmunization in Ohio's Amish: Parental fears are a greater obstacle than access to care. Pediatrics 2011;128(1): 79–84.
34. Dubé E, Laberge C, Guay M, et al. Vaccine hesitancy: An overview. Hum Vaccin Immunother 2013;9(8):1763–73.
35. Nagata JM, Isabel H-R, Anand SK, et al. Social determinants of health and seasonal influenza vaccination in adults ≥65 years: a systematic review of qualitative and quantitative data. BMC Public Health 2011;13(1):388.
36. Quinn SC. African American adults and seasonal influenza vaccination: Changing our approach can move the needle. Hum Vaccin Immunother 2018;14(3): 719–23.
37. Prins W, Butcher E, Hall LL, et al. Improving adult immunization equity: Where do the published research literature and existing resources lead? Vaccine 2017; 35(23):3020–5.
38. Freimuth VS, Jamison AM, An J, et al. Determinants of trust in the flu vaccine for African Americans and Whites. Soc Sci Med 2017;193:70–9.

39. Sevin AM, Romeo C, Gagne B, et al. Factors influencing adults' immunization practices: a pilot survey study of a diverse, urban community in central Ohio. BMC Public Health 2016;16(1). https://doi.org/10.1186/s12889-016-3107-9.
40. Luz PM, Johnson RE, Brown HE. Workplace availability, risk group and perceived barriers predictive of 2016–17 influenza vaccine uptake in the United States: A cross-sectional study. Vaccine 2017;35(43):5890–6.
41. Nowak GJ, Sheedy K, Bursey K, et al. Promoting influenza vaccination: Insights from a qualitative meta-analysis of 14 years of influenza-related communications research by U.S. Centers for Disease Control and Prevention (CDC). Vaccine 2015;33(24):2741–56.
42. Henry KA, Swiecki-Sikora AL, Stroup AM, et al. Area-based socioeconomic factors and Human Papillomavirus (HPV) vaccination among teen boys in the United States. BMC Public Health 2017;18(1):1–16.
43. Polonijo AN, Carpiano RM. Social inequalities in adolescent human papillomavirus (HPV) vaccination: a test of fundamental cause theory. Soc Sci Med 2013; 82:115–25.
44. Lu PJ, O'Halloran A, Ding H, et al. National and state-specific Td and Tdap vaccination of adult populations. Am J Prev Med 2016;50(5):616–26.
45. Douthit N, Kiv S, Dwolatzky T, Biswas S. Exposing some important barriers to health care access in the rural USA. Public Health 2015;129(6):611–20. https://doi.org/10.1016/j.puhe.2015.04.001.
46. Chan KS, Gaskin DJ, Mccleary RR, et al. Availability of Health Care Provider Offices. J Health Care Poor Underserved 2019;30(3):986–1000.
47. Hurley LP, Lindley MC, Allison MA, et al. Primary care physicians' perspective on financial issues and adult immunization in the Era of the Affordable Care Act. Vaccine 2017;35(4):647–54.
48. Iritani K. Medicare: Many Factors, Including Administrative Challenges, Affect Access to Part D Vaccinations. United States Gov Account Off. 2011;(GAO-12–61):1–97. Available at: https://www.gao.gov/products/GAO-12-61. Last Accessed June 23, 2020.
49. Stewart AM, Lindley MC, Cox MA. Medicaid provider reimbursement policy for adult immunizations. Vaccine 2015;33(43):5801–8.
50. Stewart AM, Lindley MC, Chang KHM, et al. Vaccination benefits and cost-sharing policy for non-institutionalized adult Medicaid enrollees in the United States. Vaccine 2014;32(5):618–23.
51. Bloodworth R, Chen J, Mortensen K. Variation of preventive service utilization by state Medicaid coverage, cost-sharing, and Medicaid expansion status. Prev Med (Baltim) 2018;115:97–103.
52. Walsh B, Doherty E, O'Neill C. Since the start of the vaccines for children program, uptake has increased, and most disparities have decreased. Health Aff 2016;35(2):356–64.
53. Zhou F, Shefer A, Wenger J, et al. Economic evaluation of the routine childhood immunization program in the united states, 2009. Pediatrics 2014;133(4):577–85.
54. Jacob V, Chattopadhyay SK, Hopkins DP, et al. Community Preventive Services Task Force. Increasing coverage of appropriate vaccinations: a Community Guide systematic economic review. Am J Prev Med 2016;50(6):797–808.
55. Allison MA, O'Leary ST, Lindley MC, et al. Financing of vaccine delivery in primary care practices. Acad Pediatr 2017. https://doi.org/10.1016/j.acap.2017.06.001.
56. Hurley LP, Allison MA, Dooling KL, et al. Primary care physicians' experience with zoster vaccine live (ZVL) and awareness and attitudes regarding the new recombinant zoster vaccine (RZV). Vaccine 2018;36(48):7408–14.

57. Poland GA, Hall LL, Powell JA. Effective and equitable influenza vaccine coverage in older and vulnerable adults: The need for evidence-based innovation and transformation. Vaccine 2019;37(16):2167–70.
58. Hopkins DP. Recommendation for use of immunization information systems to increase vaccination rates. J Public Health Manag Pract 2015;21(3):249–52.
59. Orenstein WA, Gellin BG, Beigi RH, et al. Recommendations from the national vaccine advisory committee: standards for adult immunization practice. Public Health Rep 2014;129(2):115–23.
60. Appel A, Everhart R, Mehler PS, et al. Lack of Ethnic Disparities in Adult Immunization Rates Among Underserved Older Patients in an Urban Public Health System. Med Care 2006;44(11):1054–8.
61. The 4 Pillars™ Practice Transformation Program for Immunization. Available at: http://www.4pillarstransformation.pitt.edu/. Last Accessed June 23, 2020.
62. Tan L. Adult vaccination: Now is the time to realize an unfulfilled potential. Hum Vaccin Immunother 2015;11(9):2158–66.
63. Maurer J, Harris KM, Uscher-Pines L. Can routine offering of influenza vaccination in office-based settings reduce racial and ethnic disparities in adult influenza vaccination? J Gen Intern Med 2014;29(12):1624–30.
64. Davis TC, Arnold C, Dillaha J, et al. Lessons learned from immunization providers: strategies for successful immunization efforts among medicare patients. NAM Perspect 2018;8(6). https://doi.org/10.31478/201806c.
65. Anandappa M, Adjei Boakye E, Li W, et al. Racial disparities in vaccination for seasonal influenza in early childhood. Public Health 2018;158:1–8.
66. Zhao Z, Smith P, Hill H. Evaluation of potentially achievable vaccination coverage with simultaneous administration of vaccines among children in the United StatesVaccine. Vaccine 2016;34(27):3030–6.
67. Lindley MC, Hurley LP, Beaty BL, et al. Vaccine financing and billing in practices serving adult patients: A follow-up survey. Vaccine 2018. https://doi.org/10.1016/j.vaccine.2018.01.015.

Immunizing in a Global Society: Vaccines for Travelers

Oritsetsemaye Otubu, MD, MPH[a,*], Ranit Mishori, MD, MHS[b]

KEYWORDS

• Travel health • Global health • Vaccine • Immunization • Vaccination
• Vaccine-preventable disease • International travel

KEY POINTS

- The risk of disease spread globally is easy with populations that are very mobile.
- International travelers are at increased risk for exposure to vaccine-preventable diseases.
- Vaccine requirements are specific to each country and to each traveler's risk.
- Unvaccinated travelers run the risk not only of becoming infected and suffering illness but also of transferring disease to the home country.
- Appropriate vaccines before travel can prevent illness to the traveler.

BACKGROUND

Global Movement

Millions of people travel internationally on any given day. More than 1.3 billion people were estimated to travel as tourists in 2017 alone.[1] According to United Nations World Tourism Organization statistics, there are 1.4 billion international travelers per year.[2] They traverse borders by foot, car, train, boat, and plane. This global movement of individuals puts millions of people at risk of contracting communicable diseases: those going into countries and regions with endemic diseases they are not immune to as well as those who may be infected serve as conduits and can introduce communicable diseases during their travel or on their return to their home country.

It is due to these risks that national, international, and transnational bodies, such as the World Health Organization (WHO), Centers for Disease Control and Prevention (CDC), and Advisory Committee on Immunization Practices (ACIP), strongly recommend travelers be fully immunized to reduce harm to individuals and communities.

Assessing Risk and Vaccine Needs/Harms

The risk of travel-related illnesses that require vaccines varies depending on destination and traveler characteristics. Individual travelers can work with a family physician

[a] Medstar Urgent Care, 1805 Columbia rd NW, Washington DC 20009, USA; [b] Department of Family Medicine, Georgetown University School of Medicine, 3900 Reservoir rd NW Washington DC 20007, USA
* Corresponding author.
E-mail address: Ogotubu@gmail.com

Prim Care Clin Office Pract 47 (2020) 497–515
https://doi.org/10.1016/j.pop.2020.05.005 primarycare.theclinics.com

or other health professional to assess their travel risk based on the diseases endemic to the region they are going to, the time of year, and the presence of acute outbreaks. In addition, travelers should discuss their own personal medical history, immunization status, purpose of their trip, and other individual risk factors.

Table 1 lists helpful resources for assessing and monitoring ongoing outbreaks and communicable disease risk by region and country.

The clinician should elicit details about the traveler's personal medical history, such as age, current pregnancy, immune deficiency, and history of allergic reactions to vaccines, to gauge the potential risk of administering travel vaccines.[3–5]

Beyond ensuring that the traveler has all the basic ACIP-recommended vaccines for age and medical history, the clinician should inquire about the purpose of the specific travel and anticipated activities and obtain a general travel history in order to make decisions about which additional vaccines may be necessary. Risks of exposure may vary by location (high-income countries vs less developed settings, urban vs rural, and climate differences), lodging (hotels in urban settings, home-stays, and outdoors), potential for animal encounters (eg, risk for rabies), and types of populations expected to be interacted with (eg, sick individuals in the case of health workers).

Table 2 lists a variety of populations of travelers and how their distinct characteristics may affect considerations for the administration of certain vaccines.

Vaccine Hesitancy and Refusal

Vaccine hesitancy and refusal also affect travelers. Common reasons to forgo vaccinations are related to cost, safety, or lack of concern of being at risk for an illness. A 2016 study reviewing data on more than 24,000 adult travelers found that the most common reason given for pretravel vaccine refusal was "a lack of concern about the associated illness."[4] Similarly, 1 large study found that parents or guardians of 30% of children in a national data set of more than 3000 children who presented for a pretravel visit refused at least 1 of the recommended travel vaccines.

SPECIFIC IMMUNIZATIONS FOR INTERNATIONAL TRAVELERS

Physicians must ensure that travelers are up to date on routine vaccines, according to ACIP recommendations, because some vaccine-preventable communicable diseases uncommonly seen in the US context, such as polio, tetanus, hepatitis A/B, measles, and meningitis, may be more prevalent in other parts of the world.

Additional vaccines are intended to cover conditions rarely seen in the US context, such as yellow fever, rabies, typhoid, cholera, and Japanese encephalitis, and should be given as indicated, based on type of travel and destination.

Table 1
Web sites for communicable disease risk and outbreak monitoring

Resource	Link
CDC	https://wwwnc.cdc.gov/travel/notices
WHO disease outbreak news	https://www.who.int/csr/don/en/
European CDC outbreak reports	https://ecdc.europa.eu/en/threats-and-outbreaks/reports-and-data
Global outbreak reports	https://outbreaks.globalincidentmap.com/
Global TravEpiNet	https://www.travelmdus.org/ https://wwwnc.cdc.gov/travel/page/gten

Table 2
Traveler type and risk

Population/Purpose	Things to Consider
Business travelers	• May spend time only in an urban setting, hotels or conference centers, or office buildings • Consider length of stay and repeat trips • Inquire about intention to stay for travel after business is done
Health workers	• Likely will come in close contact with individuals suffering from a variety of vaccine-preventable diseases • May work in rural areas or low-resource settings • May work in areas where they may encounter animals
Tourists	• Inquire about intention to visit rural areas • Inquire about intended lodging (home stays vs hotels vs hostels) • Inquire about likely contact with animals
Hikers	• May spend more time in remote and rural areas • May encounter animals • May plan on sleeping in the outdoors
Long-term expatriates	• Depending on where they are, may have a different set of vaccine schedules and requirements
Visiting friends and relatives (persons who maintain familial or other social links to a country other than that of their current citizenship or residence) Children are more likely to be visiting friends and relatives than are adults; they also are less likely to receive a pretravel consultation.[9]	• Former residents returning to their home country who may not perceive risks • One study found this group to be at increased risk of viral hepatitis, malaria, HIV, and sexually transmitted infections compared with tourists and business travelers to the same destination.
Military deployment	• Likely will follow military vaccine requirements
Scientists and researchers (eg, veterinarians and zoologists)	• May be more likely to spend a lot of time outdoors, in rural areas • May be more likely to encounter animals
Religious pilgrims (eg, hajj) and travelers to mass events (eg, Olympic games)	• Consider the population density at the destination. • Consider specific destination requirements for travel (eg, meningitis vaccine for the hajj).
Migrants (immigrants, refugees, and asylum seekers)	• Consider endemic diseases in their country of origin. • Consider immunization schedule, availability, and access in the country of origin.

The classic definition of a traveler who is visiting friends and relatives is "an immigrant returning to his country of origin for a visit with friends or relatives who is racially or ethnically distinct from the majority population in his adopted country, moving from a higher income country with low tropical disease prevalence to a lower income country with higher risk of these diseases, and who is also experiencing living conditions more similar to the local population than that of a typical tourist or business traveler."[7]

Data from Refs.[6–8]

Table 3 provides detailed information about vaccines that should be considered for international travelers. See wwwnc.cdc.gov/travel/destinations/list for the most up-to-date list of traveler vaccine recommendations.

ON THE HORIZON: VACCINES IN DEVELOPMENT

There are, of course, other communicable diseases that present a threat to international travelers, but for which there are not yet effective or commercially available vaccines.

Ebola Vaccine

Currently, only an investigational vaccine is available for the Ebola virus. Known as rVSV-ZEBOV, it was created using vesicular stomatitis virus, genetically engineered to include a component of the Zaire Ebola virus variant. It is not yet licensed but is recommended by the WHO for compassionate use, meaning for high-risk persons in areas with Ebola outbreaks caused by the Zaire strain of Ebola virus. Those at high risk include contacts of an infected patient, contacts of contacts, and health care and frontline personnel. Eligible recipients for the vaccine include children greater than 1 year old and nonpregnant adults. Adverse effects include headache, fatigue, mild fever, and myalgia. The vaccine may be protective for up to 12 months, but data currently are insufficient to determine length of protection.[35]

Malaria Vaccine

No licensed vaccine for malaria is available yet. GlaxoSmithKline developed the RTS,S vaccine, a conjugate vaccine for children ages 5 months to 17 months, which targets the malaria falciparum strain. According to the WHO, results of RTS,S phase 3 safety and efficacy trials conducted from 2009 to 2014 in 7 countries in sub-Saharan Africa showed that the vaccine generally was safe and well tolerated. It reduced, by 29%, both the number of children with severe malaria and the need for blood transfusion and, by 39%, the number of cases of malaria over 4 years of follow-up. Adverse events included febrile seizures, increased risk for meningitis, and cerebral malaria. In 2019, phase 4 trials of the vaccine began in Malawi, Kenya, and Ghana.[36]

Dengue Vaccine

The Dengvaxia vaccine is the only vaccine currently licensed for dengue fever prevention. It is a live recombinant tetravalent vaccine effective for all 4 strains of dengue virus and given as a 3-dose series, each dose 6 months apart. The vaccine efficacy at 25 months from first dose was noted to be 79% in patients seropositive for dengue infection at baseline and 38% in patients seronegative at baseline. Dengvaxia currently is approved only for use in persons ages 9 years to 45 years who have had prior laboratory-confirmed dengue infection. In May 2019, Dengvaxia was approved by the Food and Drug Administration for use in US territories (Virgin Islands, Puerto Rico, and American Samoa). Two other vaccines currently are in phase 3 trials.[37,38]

Human Immunodeficiency Virus Vaccine

No vaccine is currently licensed for use for the human immunodeficiency virus (HIV), but research and clinical trials are ongoing. In 2009, the RV144 prime-boost vaccine was found to have modest preventive effect for HIV infection in humans. In 2013, however, immunization trials were stopped due to lack of efficacy. In 2016, a new study was launched in South Africa to assess the safety and efficacy of an updated version

Table 3
Recommended travel vaccines for US residents

Vaccine	Who Needs it	What Regions of the World	Special Settings (Urban, Rural, Hiking, Working Around Animals)	When to Get it	Frequency of Boosters	Evidence of Efficacy	Potential Harms	Special Considerations; Special Populations (Children, Pregnant Women, Immune-compromised)	Procedural/ Legal Issues
Cholera vaccine	Adults 18–64 y traveling to areas of active cholera transmission	Any area with active cholera transmission—epidemic or pandemic Vaccine not routinely required by any country or territory		2 wk prior to travel	Single-dose live oral vaccine	Reduces chance of severe diarrhea by 90% at 10 d after vaccination and by 30% at 3 mo after vaccination	Hyper-sensitivity, mild gastro-intestinal symptoms	Safety in pregnancy not yet known	Only vaccine available in United States is Vaxchora, lyophilized CVD 103-HgR Not required by any country
Hepatitis A	For travelers to high risk and intermediate risk countries.	Highly endemic areas include parts of Africa and Asia; intermediate-risk areas include Central and South America, parts of Asia, and Eastern Europe; and low-risk areas include United	Rural areas and areas of low sanitation People working with nonhuman primates	Give as soon as possible before travel. Infants ages 6–11 mo can receive 1 dose prior to travel and it should not count toward their 2-dose routine vaccination (Infants <6mos should	No boosters needed with standard schedule. Accelerated schedule requires a booster dose if Twinrix is used	Immunogenicity of 1 dose of HAV is 94%–100%.	Injection site reactions, headache Hypersensitivity	Hepatitis A vaccine is considered safe to give during pregnancy. Travelers <6 mo going to countries of high-risk to intermediate-risk of endemic hepatitis A vaccine (HAV) should receive immunoglobulin prior to travel. The number of	Two monovalent intramuscular vaccines exist, Vaqta and Havrix, approved for ages 12 mo and older, given in 2 doses 6 mo apart. Twinrix, a combination intramuscular vaccine of

(*continued on next page*)

Table 3
(continued)

Vaccine	Who Needs it	What Regions of the World	Special Settings (Urban, Rural, Hiking, Working Around Animals)	When to Get it	Frequ-ency of Boosters	Evidence of Efficacy	Potential Harms	Special Considerations; Special Populations (Children, Pregnant Women, Immune-compromised)	Procedural/ Legal Issues
		States, and Western Europe		receive a single does of IGG only) Travelers ages health persons ages 12mos – 40yrs should receive 1st dose of 2 dose series as soon as possible prior to travel and receive 2nd dose 6 mo later Anyone ages >40 y, immuno-compromised, or individuals with chronic liver disease should receive HAV and also may receive immunoglobulin at the same time but at a different injection site				doses is dependent upon duration of stay in country. HAV can be used for postexposure prophylaxis (PEP) when used within 2 wk of exposure Avoid Twinrix in patients with hypersensitivity to yeast. Avoid HAV in patients with allergy to neomycin.	hepatitis A and hepatitis B, is available in the United States and equally effective for Hepatitis A and B. It is only approved for use in people 18yrs and older.

Hepatitis B	Travelers to high-risk areas. People with chronic conditions, older people, health care workers, and people who participate in high-risk activities (such as injection drug use and unprotected sex)	Africa and Western Pacific region with high prevalence of chronic hepatitis B	Travelers with high-risk behavior of unprotected sex, injection drug use Expatriates, missionaries, long-term workers in countries with high prevalence of chronic hepatitis B	Adult travelers can receive hepatitis B vaccine at least 1 mo prior to travel if using Heplisav or using an accelerated 0 d, 7 d, 21–30 d accelerated Twinrix schedule. A booster dose at 12 mo is required for the accelerated schedule.	No boosters needed for routine vaccine, only needed for accelerated schedule with Twinrix.	Overall, 3-dose series produces protective antibodies in 95% of healthy infants and >90% in healthy adults ages <40 y. Protective antibodies produced after the 2nd dose are approximately 63% in healthy infants and 75% in healthy adults <40 y.	Injection site reactions; mild systemic reactions (erythema, fever, headache, malaise); severe reactions anaphylaxis (some reports of Guillain-Barré syndrome, multiple sclerosis, optic neuritis but no demonstrable association between the disease and vaccine)	3 dose Hep B vaccines are considered safe in pregnancy. HBV also may be used for postexposure prophylaxis with hepatitis B immunoglobulin (HBIG) Avoid in persons with prior hypersensitivity to vaccine or hypersensitivity to yeast.	Four Vaccines are available in the United States. Recombivax HB is a 3 dose schedule for children and adults; Engerix-B is a 3 dose schedule vaccine for children and adults; Twinrix is a 3 dose vacicine for adults >18yrs; Heplisav-B is a 2 dose schedule for adults >18yrs. Pediarix is a combination Hep B containing vaccine used in children aged 6wks-6yrsthat but it also contains diphtheria, pertusis, polio, and tetanus so not ideal for focused Hep B immunization.

(continued on next page)

Table 3
(continued)

Vaccine	Who Needs it	What Regions of the World	Special Settings (Urban, Rural, Hiking, Working Around Animals)	When to Get it	Frequency of Boosters	Evidence of Efficacy	Potential Harms	Special Considerations; Special Populations (Children, Pregnant Women, Immune-compromised)	Procedural/Legal Issues
Influenza	Everyone ages ≥6 mo traveling to a part of the world with influenza activity and without a contra indication to the influenza vaccine.	Southern hemisphere April–September; Northern hemisphere, October-May tropics any time of year, organized tourist groups or cruise ships any time of year		2 wks prior to travel	Annual vaccine	Varies with each vaccine year. 40% effectiveness in 2017–2018 flu season	Injection site reaction- redness, soreness. h/a, myalgia, fever, malaise. Nasal spray (LAIV)[c]: URI sx, malaise, fever, myalgia, vomiting, wheezing	Contraindicated in persons with previous severe allergic reaction to influenza vaccine Children ages 6mos to 8yrs require 2 doses of influenza vaccine 4 weeks apart if they have never received 2 doses of trivalent or quadrivalent influenza vaccine >4weeks apart. Live attenuated vaccine should not be used in pregnancy or immuno-compromised persons.	Influenza strains in northern and southern hemispheres may be different. If traveling from one region to the other and strains are different, both vaccines are necessary. Several approved flu vaccines are available and the selection is updated annually with each flu season. Trivalent and quadrivalent vaccines exist as inactivated influenza vaccine (IIV) or Live Attenuated Ifluenza vaccine (LAIV). Please check for updates on the

Japanese encephalitis	Age >2mos traveling to areas endemic with Japanese Encephalitis.	Most of Asia and Western Pacific	Mostly in rural and agricultural areas. Occasionally in urban areas. Longer duration of travel also increases risk	7 d prior to travel	Standard dosing is 2 doses of Ixiaro vaccine 28 d apart. Accelerated primary dosing is 2 doses 7 d apart. A booster dose is recommended for adults and children ≥ 1 yr after primary dose for travelers with ongoing exposure.	No efficacy data exist. Protectiveness of vaccine has been evaluated based on persistence of seroprotective neutralizing antibodies. Studies show waning amount of protection from 83% at 6 mo to 48% at 24 mo after 1st dose of 2-dose series. Increased seroprotection to 98% at 12 mo after booster dose given at 15 mo after 1st dose of 2-dose series. Decreased immunogenicity in adults ≥65yrs.	Injection site reaction. Fever, headache, urticarial rash. Hypersensitivity	No studies have been done to determine safety and efficacy in pregnant women.	Ixiaro, an inactivated vaccine, is the only vaccine available for use in the U.S
Measles Mumps Rubella	Children age >6mos and adults who have not received the vaccine	Globally, except Antarctica		Be fully vaccinated at least 2 weeks prior to departure. For children ages 6-11 mos give 1 dose before travel for Measles protection and then	no booster required	Effectiveness against measles is 85% if one dose is given at age 9mos and 93% if given at 1yr or later. One dose is 78% and 97% effective against rubella	Anaphylaxis, thrombocytopenia, arthralgias, febrile seizures	Do not give to immunosuppressed. Should be given on same day or 4 wk before or after other live vaccines like yellow fever. Do not give in pregnancy.	Live attenuated vaccine available as MMR and MMRV in the U.S

(continued on next page)

Table 3 (*continued*)

Vaccine	Who Needs it	What Regions of the World	Special Settings (Urban, Rural, Hiking, Working Around Animals)	When to Get it	Frequency of Boosters	Evidence of Efficacy	Potential Harms	Special Considerations; Special Populations (Children, Pregnant Women, Immune-compromised)	Procedural/ Legal Issues
				follow standard schedule not counting travel dose. For children ages 12-15mos give 2 doses 4 weeks apart prior to travel.		and mumps respectively. 2 doses confer effectiveness of 97% against measles and 88% against mumps Post exposure prophylaxis with MMR may be beneficial for measles prevention if obtained within 72hrs of exposure.			
Meningitis	All travelers ages 2 mo – 55 y going to high-risk countries. Need coverage against serotype A	High-risk areas include countries in the meningitis belt of sub-Saharan Africa, which includes parts of Guinea Bissau, Gambia, Senegal, Burkina Faso, Cote d'Ivoire, Ghana, Benin, Nigeria, Niger, Mali, Mauritania, Chad,		At least 10 d prior to travel A protective antibody response is within 10 d of vaccination Age 2mos at start of series requires 4 doses at age 2mo, 4mo, 6mo, 12mos using Menveo vaccine. Age 7-23 mos at start of series requires a 2 dose regimen >3mos	Every 3–5 y if individual continues to be in high-risk area	Vaccine effectiveness was 79% in adolescents at <1yr postvaccinaton. Protection wanes over time.	Injection site reaction, malaise, headache	According to the CDC, outbreaks of meningococcal disease have been associated with hajj pilgrimage to Saudi Arabia. Pregnant women can receive the MenACWY vaccine	Proof of tetravalent vaccine required for travel by Saudi Arabia for pilgrims and guest workers 4 vaccines avaialbe in U.S. Menveo and Menactra are both tetravalent vaccines covering serogroups ACWY and can be used for children and adults. Trumenba and Bexsero cover serogroup B

		Cameroon, Central African Republic, Sudan, South Sudan, Ethiopia, Eritrea, Uganda, Kenya, and Democratic Republic of Congo	apart and minimum of 8wks apart if limited time before travel. Age >2yrs need at least 1 dose of quadrivalent vaccine before travel Children receiving meningococcal vaccine for travel prior to age 10 will still need to follow the routine schedule and get additional vaccines at age 10-11yrs and at age 16yrs.					only and generally recommended for use in age 10–25yrs.
Polio	All travelers to areas of active polio transmission	Afghanistan, Pakistan, Nigeria	Depends on vaccination status at time of travel but generally between 4weeks and 12 months before departure date. Children should get the vaccine at 2mo, 4 mos, 6-18 mos. If limited time then IPV dosing for infants should be: 1st dose >6wks, 2nd and 3rd dose given >;4wks after previous dose, 4th dose >6mos after 3rd dose. If pressed for time in adult with no prior vaccination,	Booster at age 4-6yrs for child who received childhood series. Series given in childhood and 1 time booster for adults who completed series Vaccination for	Completion of 3-dose series confers lifetime immunity.	Minor injection site reaction IPV contains streptomycin, neomycin, and polymyxin B; so avoid in patients with allergy to these medications. OPV can cause vaccine derived polio virus.	IPV can be administered during pregnancy and lactation and to immuno -compromised persons using adult guidelines.	A new OPV that covers type 2 poliovirus is being investigated. Inactivated Polio Vaccine is the only polio vaccine available in U.S currently Long-term travelers and residents traveling from countries with active polio transmission may need to show proof of vaccination.

(continued on next page)

Table 3
(*continued*)

Vaccine	Who Needs it	What Regions of the World	Special Settings (Urban, Rural, Hiking, Working Around Animals)	When to Get it	Frequency of Boosters	Evidence of Efficacy	Potential Harms	Special Considerations; Special Populations (Children, Pregnant Women, Immune-compromised)	Procedural/ Legal Issues
				Alternative Adult IPV dosing: 3 doses 4 weeks apart.	Unvaccinated or incompletely vaccinated adults depends on time available before travel. If at least 8 wk, then give 3 doses IPV 4 wk apart; if <8 wk but >4 wk, then give 2 doses 4 wk apart; if <4 wk prior to travel, then 1 dose IPV should be given.				

rabies	Travelers going to rabies enzootic areas	South and Central America, Africa, and Asia	Working with animals/wildlife, visiting remote areas, and working in a rabies lab.	At least 3 wk before travel Don't immunize if 3 dose series can't be completed before travel	Booster not required for persons who completed 3 dose series but may require postexposure prophylaxis if exposed	99% effective when used for post exposure prophylaxis	Include local reaction at the site of vaccination, including erythema, pain, itching, or mild systemic reactions of nausea, abdominal pain, muscle aches, headache, dizziness	Vaccine should be given in the deltoid muscle only. Vaccine is used for pre-exposure and postexposure. Dosing for post exposure prophylaxis is based on preexposure prophylaxis status. Safe to give in Pregnancy	2 vaccines available in the U.S: Imovax (human diploid cell culture vaccine, HDCV)and Rabavert (purified chick embryo cell culture, PCEC) are both inactivated vaccines.
Tetanus	All travelers are recommended to receive the 3-dose tetanus vaccine series if not previously vaccinated.	Risk is worldwide.	Rural and agricultural areas where contact with animal excreta or soil contaminated with it is more likely	If no prior history of tetanus vaccine, need 3 dose series. Tdap as 1st dose, followed by 2nd dose of Td or Tdap 4weeks later, then 3rd dose of tdap or td 6 months after 2nd dose.	A booster is needed every 10 y for anyone with complete series. People with incomplete vaccine record should receive catch-up doses and then boosters every 10 y.	TdaP, Td, and DtaP confer 95% protective levels of diphtheria antitoxin, and 100% protective levels for tetanus antitoxin. Acellular pertussis protects 73%–85% of those vaccinated. Protection decreases over time, hence the need for boosters. (28)	Local injection-site reactions Hypersensitivity	Due to the increasing incidence of pertussis infection in the United States, TdaP is recommended as part of the series or as a booster in previously vaccinated individuals. The WHO recommends diphtheria-containing vaccines rather than tetanus toxoid alone. Safe in pregnancy and lactation	DTAP vaccines in US: Daptacel, Pinrix, Kinrix, Quatracel, Pentacel, Pediarix Tdap vaccines in US: Adacel, Boostrix TD vaccines in US: Tenivax, Generic Td DT vaccines in US: Generic DT

(continued on next page)

Table 3
(continued)

Vaccine	Who Needs it	What Regions of the World	Special Settings (Urban, Rural, Hiking, Working Around Animals)	When to Get it	Frequency of Boosters	Evidence of Efficacy	Potential Harms	Special Considerations; Special Populations (Children, Pregnant Women, Immune-compromised)	Procedural/ Legal Issues
Tick-borne encephalitis	Travellers to parts of Europe and Asia	Europe and Asia; from Eastern France to Northern Japan and from Northern Russia to Albania	Most cases occur April–November. High risk in forested areas. Negligible risk in urban unforested areas.	Vaccine not available in the U.S	Booster dose every 3 y for those at continued risk of exposure.	99% in regularly vaccinated persons after the 2nd dose, 95% in persons with record of irregular vaccination	Local injection site reaction hypersensitivity	Avoid ingestion of unpasteurized dairy products	Inactivated cell culture derived vaccines are available in Europe
Typhoid	Travelers to countries with high-risk for infection	High-risk areas include Southern Asia (primarily India, Pakistan, and Bangladesh), Africa and Southeast Asia. Lower-risk areas include East Asia, South America, and the Caribbean.		At least 2 wk before travel	Every 2 y for IM vaccine if individual remains in high-risk area Every 5 y for oral vaccine if remains in high-risk area	Both oral and intramuscular vaccines provide a 50%–80% level of protection.	IM vaccine: fever, h/a, injection site reaction Oral vaccine: fever, h/a, stomach pain, nausea, vomiting	Antibiotics should not be taken 3 d before or after the administration of the oral vaccine. Inactivated IM vaccine for ages ≥2 y Live attenuated oral vaccine for ages ≥6 y	Two uncongugated Typhoid vaccines available US: vivotif (Oral live attenuate vaccine) and a Vi capsular, polysacharide vaccine

Yellow fever	Travelers 9 mo and older going to or through high-risk countries	High-risk countries in sub-Saharan Africa and South America		10 d before travel	No longer recom-mended for routine travelers because vaccine confers lifetime immunity. A booster may be consi-dered in select groups, including persons in high-risk setting 10 y after initial dose.	Seroconversion of >90% at 10 d after immunization	Headache, myalgia, fever, anaphylaxis	Precaution in pregnant and immunocom-promised	Not all countries have adopted the no booster recommendation. Check CDC travel site before traveling.

Abbreviations: IIV, inactivated influenza vaccine; LAIV, live attenuated influenza vaccine; RIV, recombinant influenza vaccineHBIG- hep B immunoglobulin; HBV, hepatitis B vaccine; IM, intramuscular; MMR, measles mumps rubella; MMRV, meases mump rubella vaccine; OPV, oral polio virus; Sx, symptom; TD =Tetanus Diphtheria, Tdap, Tetanus, Diphterhea, acelluar Pertusis, URI, upper respiratory Infection.

Data from Refs.[10–34]

of RT144 vaccine in adults. Other vaccines are being researched, including VCR01 antibody intravenous infusion and a mosaic vaccine.[39]

PRACTICAL ISSUES

Obtaining Travel Vaccines

Travel vaccines are not always available at primary care offices. If needed, clinicians may refer patients to obtain their travel vaccines in health departments or specialized travel clinics. A global directory of travel clinics can be found at https://www.istm.org/AF_CstmClinicDirectory.asp.

Documentation

Once vaccines have been administered, documentation is important, especially because some countries may require evidence of immunization in the form of certificates. For example, certain countries require that travelers present proof of yellow fever administration, so clinicians should make sure they can provide patients with a signed and stamped yellow card or International Certificate of Vaccination or Prophylaxis.[40] Saudi Arabian authorities require proof of meningitis immunization for all travelers attending the annual hajj.[41] It is advisable in general to provide patients a printout of their entire immunization record.

Cost

Visits to travel clinics may be costly and depend on a variety of factors, including the number of vaccines needed. Most health insurance programs do not cover travel-related immunizations, and it is important to advise patients that the vaccines are expensive. Many specialty travel clinics post the costs online. For example, a yellow fever vaccine can cost close to $200, a typhoid injection approximately $100, Japanese encephalitis vaccine approximately $300 per shot (2 are needed), and rabies vaccines can cost approximately $350 per shot (3 needed); and these are on top of the cost of an evaluation by a licensed medical professional (physician or nurse).[42]

SUMMARY

In an increasingly global world, where millions travel internationally daily, immunizations are 1 tool to protect the health of the individual traveler and the community. Primary care physicians should discuss travel plans with their patients, helping them identify any necessary immunizations or prophylaxis prior to leaving. Using resources from the WHO and CDC can facilitate these conversations, making it easier for busy clinicians to provide up-to-date and accurate advice.

DISCLOSURE

The authors have nothing to disclose.

REFERENCES

1. International tourism, number of arrivals. The world bank website. Available at: https://data.worldbank.org/indicator/ST.INT.ARVL?end=2017&start=2017&view=bar. Accessed September 26, 2019.
2. Roser M. Tourism. *Our World in Data*.org. 2019. Available at: https://ourworldindata.org/tourism. Accessed September 26, 2019.

3. Hagmann S, LaRocque RC, Rao SR, et al. Pre-travel health preparation of pediatric international travelers: analysis from the Global TravEpiNet Consortium. J Pediatric Infect Dis Soc 2012;2(4):327–34.
4. Hendel-Paterson B, Swanson SJ. Pediatric travelers visiting friends and relatives (VFR) abroad: illnesses, barriers and pre-travel recommendations. Travel Med Infect Dis 2011;9(4):192–203.
5. Matteelli A, Carvalho ACC, Bigoni S. Visiting relatives and friends (VFR), pregnant, and other vulnerable travelers. Infect Dis Clin North Am 2012;26(3):625–35.
6. Chen LH, Leder K, Wilson ME. Business travelers: vaccination considerations for this population. Expert Rev Vaccines 2013;12(4):453–66.
7. Barnett ED, MacPherson DW, Stauffer WM, et al. The visiting friends or relatives traveler in the 21st century: time for a new definition. J Travel Med 2010;17(3):163–70.
8. Fenner L, Weber R, Steffen R, et al. Imported infectious disease and purpose of travel, Switzerland. Emerg Infect Dis 2007;13(2). https://doi.org/10.3201/eid1302.060847.
9. Lammert SM, Rao SR, Jentes ES, et al. Refusal of recommended travel-related vaccines among U.S. international travellers in Global TravEpiNet. J Travel Med 2016;24(1). https://doi.org/10.1093/jtm/taw075.
10. Cholera-Vibrio Cholera infection: vaccines. Center for disease control and prevention website. Available at: https://www.cdc.gov/cholera/vaccines.html. Accessed September 30, 2019.
11. Centers for Disease Control and Prevention. CDC yellow book 2018: health information for International Travel. New York: Oxford University Press; 2017. Available at: https://wwwnc.cdc.gov/travel/yellowbook/2020/travel-related-infectious-diseases/hepatitis-a#table402. Accessed September 23, 2019.
12. Nelson NP, Link-Gelles L, Hofmeister MG, et al. Update: recommendations of the Advisory Committee on Immunization Practices for Use of Hepatitis A Vaccine for Postexposure Prophylaxis and for Preexposure Prophylaxis for International Travel. MMWR Morb Mortal Wkly Rep 2018;67(43):1216–20. Available at: https://www.cdc.gov/mmwr/volumes/67/wr/mm6743a5.htm?s_cid=mm6743a5_e. Accessed September 23, 2019.
13. Ask the experts: Hepatitis A. Immunization Action Coalition website. Available at: https://www.immunize.org/askexperts/experts_hepa.asp. Accessed September 23, 2019.
14. Centers for Disease Control and Prevention. CDC yellow book 2018: health information for international travel. New York: Oxford University Press; 2017. Available at: https://wwwnc.cdc.gov/travel/yellowbook/2020/travel-related-infectious-diseases/hepatitis-b. Accessed September 23, 2019.
15. Schilie S, Velozzi Z, Reginald V, et al. Prevention of Hepatitis B Virus Infection in the United States: recommendations of the Advisory Committee on Immunization Practices. MMWR Morb Mortal Wkly Rep 2018;67(1):1–31. Available at: https://www.cdc.gov/mmwr/volumes/67/rr/rr6701a1.htm?s_cid=rr6701a1_e. Accessed September 24, 2019.
16. Grohskopf LA, Sokolow LZ, Broder KR, et al. Prevention and control of influenza vaccines: recommendations of Advisory committee on immunization practices – United States 2016-17 influenza vaccine. MMWR Morb Mortal Wkly Rep 2016;65(5):1–64. Available at: https://www.cdc.gov/mmwr/volumes/65/rr/rr6505a1.htm?s_cid=rr6505a1_w#influenza_vaccination_persons_history_egg_allergy. Accessed September 23, 2019.

17. Hills S, Walter EB, Atmar RL, et al. Japanese encephalitis vaccines: recommendations of the advisory committee on immunization practices. MMWR Morb Mortal Wkly Rep 2019;68(2):1–33. Available at: https://www.cdc.gov/mmwr/volumes/68/rr/rr6802a1.htm?s_cid=rr6802a1_x. Accessed September 23, 2019.
18. Centers for Disease Control and Prevention. CDC yellow book 2018: health information for international travel. New York: Oxford University Press; 2017. Available at: https://wwwnc.cdc.gov/travel/yellowbook/2020/travel-related-infectious-diseases/japanese-encephalitis#map407. Accessed September 23, 2019.
19. Centers for Disease Control and Prevention. CDC yellow book 2018: health information for international travel. New York: Oxford University Press; 2017. Available at: https://wwwnc.cdc.gov/travel/yellowbook/2020/travel-related-infectious-diseases/measles-rubeola. Accessed September 23, 2019.
20. Centers for Disease Control and Prevention. CDC yellow book 2018: health information for international travel. New York: Oxford University Press; 2017. Available at: https://wwwnc.cdc.gov/travel/yellowbook/2020/travel-related-infectious-diseases/mumps. Accessed September 23, 2019.
21. Centers for Disease Control and Prevention. CDC yellow book 2018: health information for international travel. New York: Oxford University Press; 2017. Available at: https://wwwnc.cdc.gov/travel/yellowbook/2020/travel-related-infectious-diseases/rubella. Accessed September 23, 2019.
22. Centers for Disease Control and Prevention. CDC yellow book 2018: health information for international travel. New York: Oxford University Press; 2017. Available at: https://wwwnc.cdc.gov/travel/yellowbook/2020/travel-related-infectious-diseases/meningococcal-disease. Accessed September 23, 2019.
23. Measles, Mumps, Rubella Vaccines: what everyone should know. Center for Disease Control Website. Available at https://www.cdc.gov/vaccines/vpd/mmr/public/. Accessed June 18, 2020.
24. Cohn AC, MacNeil JR, Harrison LH, et al. Effectiveness and duration of protection of one dose of meningococcal conjugate vaccine. Pediatrics 2017;139(2). https://doi.org/10.1542/peds.2016-2193.
25. Centers for Disease Control and Prevention. CDC yellow book 2018: health information for international travel. New York: Oxford University Press; 2017. Available at: https://wwwnc.cdc.gov/travel/yellowbook/2020/travel-related-infectious-diseases/poliomyelitis. Accessed September 23, 2019.
26. Centers for Disease Control and Prevention. CDC yellow book 2018: health information for international travel. New York: Oxford University Press; 2017. Available at: https://wwwnc.cdc.gov/travel/yellowbook/2020/travel-related-infectious-diseases/rabies#table416. Accessed September 23, 2019.
27. World Health Organization. Rabies vaccines: WHO position paper. Wkly Epidemiol Rec 2018;16(93):201–20. Available at: https://apps.who.int/iris/bitstream/handle/10665/272371/WER9316.pdf?ua=1. Accessed September 23, 2019.
28. Ask the experts: Tetanus. Immunization Action Coalition website. Available at: https://www.immunize.org/askexperts/experts_per.asp. Accessed September 23, 2019.
29. Centers for Disease Control and Prevention. CDC yellow book 2018: health information for international travel. New York: Oxford University Press; 2017. Available at: https://wwwnc.cdc.gov/travel/yellowbook/2020/travel-related-infectious-diseases/tetanus. Accessed September 23, 2019.
30. Tetanus Q&A. Immunization Action Coalition website. Available at: https://www.immunize.org/catg.d/p4220.pdf. Accessed September 23, 2019.

31. About Diphtheria, Tetanus, and Pertusis Vaccines. Center for Disease control website. Available at: https://www.cdc.gov/vaccines/vpd/dtap-tdap-td/hcp/about-vaccine.html. Accessed June 18, 2020.
32. Tick Borne Encephalitis. Center for Disease control website. Available at: https://wwwnc.cdc.gov/travel/diseases/tickborne-encephalitis. Accessed June 18, 2020.
33. Yellow fever vaccine recommendations. Center for Disease Control and Prevention website. Available at: https://www.cdc.gov/yellowfever/vaccine/vaccine-recommendations.html. Accessed September 23, 2019.
34. Yellow fever vaccine package insert. Food and Drug Administration. [PDF file]. Available at: https://www.fda.gov/media/76015/download. Accessed September 23, 2019.
35. Ebola vaccine frequently asked questions. World Health Organization website. 2018. Available at: https://www.who.int/emergencies/diseases/ebola/frequently-asked-questions/ebola-vaccine. Accessed September 23, 2019.
36. Q&A on malaria vaccine implementation programme. World Health Organization website. 2019. Available at: https://www.who.int/malaria/media/malaria-vaccine-implementation-qa/en/. Accessed September 23, 2019.
37. Dengue vaccines. Center for disease control and prevention website. Available at: https://www.cdc.gov/dengue/prevention/dengue-vaccine.html. Accessed September 23, 2019.
38. Centers for Disease Control and Prevention. CDC yellow book 2018: health information for international travel. New York: Oxford University Press; 2017. Available at: https://wwwnc.cdc.gov/travel/yellowbook/2020/travel-related-infectious-diseases/dengue. Accessed September 23, 2019.
39. History of HIV Vaccine Research. National Institute of Allergy and Infectious diseases. 2018. Available at: https://www.niaid.nih.gov/diseases-conditions/hiv-vaccine-research-history. Accessed September 25, 2019.
40. Country list: yellow fever vaccination requirements and recommendations; malaria situation; and other vaccination requirements. World Health Organization website. Available at: https://www.who.int/ith/ITH_country_list.pdf?ua=1. Accessed September 27, 2019.
41. Visa application:Hajj and Umrah health requirements. Embassy of the kingdom of Saudi Arabia website. Available at: https://www.saudiembassy.net/hajj-and-umrah-health-requirements. Accessed September 27, 2019.
42. Pricing structure. The Washington Travel Clinic website. Available at: https://www.washingtontravelclinic.com/pricing/. Accessed September 27, 2019.

What's New in Vaccine Science

Margot Savoy, MD, MPH, CPE, CMQ

KEYWORDS

• Vaccine • Immunization • Vaccine science • Adjuvant • Microneedle • Immunotherapy

KEY POINTS

- Adjuvants are vaccine components used to enhance the immunogenicity of immunizations and advances in development have enabled researchers to develop increasingly effective vaccines.
- Advances in vaccine delivery systems include using smaller needles, patches, air gun, and alternative site options for delivering immunizations in more comfortable, effective, and acceptable ways.
- Vaccines will continue prevent infectious diseases but new applications can include preventing cancer and treating diseases, such as type 1 diabetes, multiple sclerosis, and asthma.

INTRODUCTION

Protecting humans from infections by artificially inducing immunity has been a medical practice since at least the tenth century. **Table 1** describes common practices for inducing immunity. Inoculation and variolation to induce immunity against smallpox was used widely in China, Turkey, India, Ethiopia, and West African countries.[1] Although one typically thinks of the history of vaccination beginning with Dr Edward Jenner, Dr Benjamin Jesty was the first to document use of cowpox to prevent smallpox disease; however, Dr Edward Jenner is credited with using scientific rigor to understand the process and lay the foundation for future immunology advances.[2–5]

Today vaccines can provide immunity against and treatment of a growing number of diseases including noninfectious conditions. As shown in **Table 2**, vaccines are created from attenuated (weakened or killed) forms of the virus or bacteria, surface proteins expressed by the microorganism, or even the toxin itself.

Vaccine science continues to evolve allowing access to more effective vaccines with improved side effect profiles, and expanding opportunities for use not only in prevention of infectious and noninfectious disease but also in disease treatment.

Family & Community Medicine, Temple Faculty Practice, Lewis Katz School of Medicine at Temple University, 1316 West Ontario Street, Room 310, Philadelphia, PA 19140, USA
E-mail address: Margot.Savoy@tuhs.temple.edu

Prim Care Clin Office Pract 47 (2020) 517–528
https://doi.org/10.1016/j.pop.2020.05.006 **primarycare.theclinics.com**

Table 1 Common methods for inducing immunity	
Inoculation	Introduction of an antigenic substance or vaccine into the body to produce immunity to a specific disease Injection of the variola virus taken from a pustule or scab of a smallpox sufferer into the superficial layers of the skin
Variolation	Inoculating the smallpox virus itself into the skin
Vaccination	Treatment with a vaccine to produce immunity against a disease; inoculation
Immunization	The process by which an individual's immune system becomes fortified against an agent (known as the immunogen), typically through inoculation

Data from Refs.[1–4]

ADVANCES IN ADJUVANT TECHNOLOGY

Adjuvants are additives used to help boost the immune response to a vaccine. Adjuvants are typically pathogen components, particulates, or a combination of the two. The first adjuvants, aluminum salts, were used beginning in the 1930s to enhance diphtheria and tetanus vaccines. Until 2009, alum was the only available adjuvant in the United States. As technology has improved, so have the available adjuvants. More recent adjuvants improve immunity by targeting key areas of the immune system.[6–8] Current Food and Drug Administration (FDA) licensed adjuvanted vaccines in the United States are shown in **Table 3**.

Hepatitis B

Hepatitis B is a viral infection that can cause chronic infection, cirrhosis, and liver cancer. It is transmitted through mucosal or percutaneous contact with infected blood or

Table 2
Types of vaccines

Type	Vaccine Is Created from	Examples
Live-attenuated	Weakened type of the virus	Measles, mumps, rubella Rotavirus Smallpox Varicella Yellow fever
Inactivated	Killed version of the bacteria/virus	Hepatitis A Influenza (injection) Polio (injection) Rabies
Subunit, recombinant, polysaccharide and conjugate	Pieces of the bacteria/virus, such as a surface protein, sugar, or capsid	*Haemophilus influenzae b* Hepatitis B Human papillomavirus Pertussis Pneumococcal disease Meningococcal disease Varicella (shingles)
Toxoid	Toxin produced by the bacteria/virus	Diphtheria Tetanus

Data from Hamilton JL. Vaccine science and immunology. In: Rockwell P, editor. Vaccine science and immunization guideline: a practical guide for primary care. Cham, Switzerland: Springer; 2017.

Table 3
FDA-licensed adjuvanted vaccines in the United States

Adjuvant		Vaccines
Aluminum	Aluminum salts	Anthrax, DT, DTaP (Daptacel), DTaP (Infanrix), DTaP-IPV (Kinrix), DTaP-IPV (Quadracel), DTaP-HepB-IPV (Pediarix), DTaP –IPV/Hib (Pentacel), Hep A (Havrix), Hep A (Vaqta), Hep B (Engerix-B), Hep B (Recombivax), HepA/Hep B (Twinrix), HIB (PedvaxHIB), HPV (Gardasil 9), Japanese encephalitis (Ixiaro), MenB (Bexsero, Trumenba), Pneumococcal (Prevnar 13), Td (Tenivac), Td (Mass Biologics), Tdap (Adacel), Tdap (Boostrix)
AS04	Combination of alum and monophosphoryl lipid A, an immune-stimulating lipid (fat) isolated from the surface of bacteria	Cervarix
MF59	Oil in water emulsion composed of squalene, which is a naturally occurring oil found in many plant and animal cells, and in humans	Fluad
$AS01_B$	Monophosphoryl lipid A, an immune-boosting substance isolated from the surface of bacteria, and QS-21, a natural compound extracted from the Chilean soapbark tree (*Quillaja saponaria* Molina)	Shingrix
CpG 1018	Cytosine phosphoguanine motifs, which is a synthetic form of DNA that mimics bacterial and viral genetic material	Heplisav-B

Data from Centers for Disease Control and Prevention. Vaccine safety common concerns. Available at: https://www.cdc.gov/vaccinesafety/concerns/adjuvants.html; and Didierlaurent AM, Morel S, Lockman L, et,al. AS04, an aluminum salt- and TLR4 agonist-based adjuvant system, induces a transient localized innate immune response leading to enhanced adaptive immunity. J Immunol. 2009;183(10):6186–97.

bodily fluids. The first vaccine against hepatitis B was developed in 1975 from a heat-treated form of the virus. A commercially available version of the vaccine was introduced in 1982. Hepatax (Merck) was a plasma-derived vaccine created from formaldehyde and heat-inactivated viral particles extracted from the blood of infected donors. In 1986 the first DNA recombinant hepatitis B vaccine was licensed offering improved immunogenicity and eliminating the risk of contracting hepatitis B from the vaccine. In 2018 a new vaccine, Heplisav-B, was licensed. All four hepatitis B vaccines use the same recombinant yeast-derived hepatitis surface antigen with an immunostimulatory adjuvant. Although Engerix-B, Recombivax HB, and Twinrix each use aluminum hydroxide, Heplisav-B uses a new synthetic oligonucleotide immunostimulatory adjuvant developed from a synthetic form of DNA that mimics bacterial and viral genetic material. Synthetic cytosine phosphoguanine stimulated the immune system by activating the toll-like receptor 9 pathway, which induces cytokine production (includes interleukin-12 and interferon-α). In three randomized, observer-blinded trials two doses (0 and 4 weeks) of Heplisav-B achieved significantly higher seroprotection rates than three doses (0, 1, and 6 months) of Engerix-B. Both vaccines' seroprotection decreases with age, and the rates remained significantly higher following Heplisav-B compared with Engerix-B.[9–12]

Varicella (Zoster)

Herpes zoster (shingles) is a reactivation of a dormant varicella virus in the dorsal root ganglion. Typically it causes a painful, vesicular rash along a dermatome. The first vaccine to prevent herpes zoster, zoster vaccine live (ZVL; Zostavax), is a live attenuated vaccine delivered in one dose. Licensed in 2006 in the United States, the vaccine reduced the risk of developing shingles by 51% and postherpetic neuralgia by 67%.[13,14] In 2017 a new vaccine, zoster vaccine recombinant, adjuvanted (RZV, Shingrix), two-dose, subunit vaccine containing recombinant glycoprotein E in combination with a novel adjuvant (AS01B) was licensed by the FDA. AS01B is comprised of monophosphoryl lipid A, which is isolated from the surface of bacteria, and QS-21, a natural compound extracted from the Chilean soapbark tree (*Quillaja saponaria* Molina). RZV outperformed ZVL in immune response and duration of protection, leading the Advisory Committee on Immunization Practices to not only recommend RZV preferentially but to recommend revaccination of those who previously received ZVL.[15–17]

VACCINE DELIVERY SYSTEM ADVANCES

Vaccinations have traditionally been administered as an intramuscular or subcutaneous hypodermic injection or via an oral route. These vaccines typically work by inducing serum IgG responses and inducing T-cell responses in the bloodstream. Needle-free technologies leveraging skin and mucosal surfaces are attractive sites for noninvasive vaccine delivery and offer unique immunologic responses including IgA induction.[18]

MUCOSAL DELIVERY

The mucosal immune system provides the first line of defense protecting the body against pathogens that attempt to enter through the respiratory tract, intestines, and urogenital tract. The mucosal immune system leverages a combination of barrier methods, IgA, and mucosal-associated lymphoid tissue.[19–21] Vaccines that are able to leverage the mucosal system are not dependent on the bloodstream T-cell pathway, expanding options for novel vaccines against infectious agents and cancers that could be used across populations including those with T-cell deficiencies.

Mucosal vaccine administration options include intranasal, intratracheal, oral, intrarectal, sublingual, intravaginal, and intraocular routes. Most currently available vaccines are oral. There are commercially available mucosal vaccines in the United States against adenovirus, poliovirus, *Vibrio cholerae*, *Salmonella typhi*, rotavirus, and influenza. **Table 4** lists the current licensed mucosal vaccines in the United States. Clinical trials continue to explore new mucosal vaccines for *Bordetella pertussis*, enterotoxigenic *Escherichia coli*, *V cholerae*, *Shigella sonnei*, and norovirus in addition to cancer vaccines against colon, lung, head and neck, and genital tumors.[20]

The first commercially available intranasal vaccine licensed in the United States was the live attenuated influenza vaccine (Flumist) in 2003.[22,23] Based on a flu strain that has low virulence and replicates poorly at body temperature, live attenuated influenza vaccine primarily stimulates the production of mucosal IgA but is also thought to stimulate systemic IgG, and T cells in healthy adults and children.[23]

Table 4
Mucosal vaccines licensed for use in the United States

Manufacturer	Proper Name	Trade Name	Indication
Oral			
Barr Labs, Inc	Adenovirus type 4 and type 7 vaccine, live, oral	n/a	Indicated for active immunization for the prevention of febrile acute respiratory disease caused by adenovirus type 4 and type 7
Pax Vax Bermuda Ltd	Cholera vaccine live oral	Vaxchora	Indicated for use in adults 18 through 64 y of age traveling to cholera-affected areas for active immunization against disease cause by *Vibrio cholera* serogroup
GlaxoSmithKline Biologicals	Rotavirus vaccine, live, oral	Rotarix	For the prevention of rotavirus gastroenteritis caused by G1 and non-G1 types (G3, G4, and G9), for use in infants 6–24 wk of age
Merck & Co, Inc	Rotavirus vaccine, live, oral, pentavalent	RotaTeq	For prevention of rotavirus gastroenteritis in infants 6–32 wk of age caused by types G1, G2, G3, G4, and G9
Berna Biotech, Ltd	Typhoid vaccine live oral ty21a	Vivotif	For immunization of adults and children >6 y of age against disease caused by *Salmonella typhi*
Intranasal			
MedImmune, LLC	Influenza vaccine live, intranasal	FluMist	For the active immunization of individuals 2–49 y of age against influenza disease caused by influenza virus subtypes A and type B contained in the vaccine
MedImmune, LLC	Influenza vaccine live, intranasal	FluMist Quadrivalent	For active immunization of individuals 2 through 49 y of age for the prevention of influenza disease caused by influenza A subtype viruses and type B viruses contained in the vaccine

Adapted from Federal Drug Administration. Vaccines licensed for use in the United States. *n/a*, not applicable. Available at: https://www.fda.gov/vaccines-blood-biologics/vaccines/vaccines-licensed-use-united-states.

SKIN DELIVERY

Transdermal patches deliver medications by applying a formulation that permeates the skin ultimately delivering the medication to the bloodstream. Mechanisms to penetrate the stratum corneum include abrasion, thermal ablation, electricity, and microneedles.[24–26] **Fig. 1** shows the depth of vaccine delivery by mechanism.

Abrasion

Increasing the skin's permeability by applying a topical abrasive agent to the stratum corneum before applying the target medication enhances the absorption of the medication.[27] Commonly used in cosmetic dermatology applications, some believe that the mechanism could be used to deliver other therapeutics through the stratum corneum including vaccines.

Electricity

Although neither is available commercially, iontophoresis and electroporation leverage electricity to successfully deliver vaccines transdermally.[28] Electroporation disrupts cellular membranes to allow transfer of the vaccine, whereas iontophoresis leverages electrostatic effects to drive the vaccine through the skin. These methods have been limited by side effects including burns, scars, and pain.[29]

Microneedle

Use of bifurcated needles to repeatedly puncture the dermis has successfully delivered live smallpox vaccination.[30] In the 1990s advances in microneedle technology provided a novel way to bypass the stratum corneum layer and deliver medications to the dermis. Microneedles are used alone or in combination with application of an

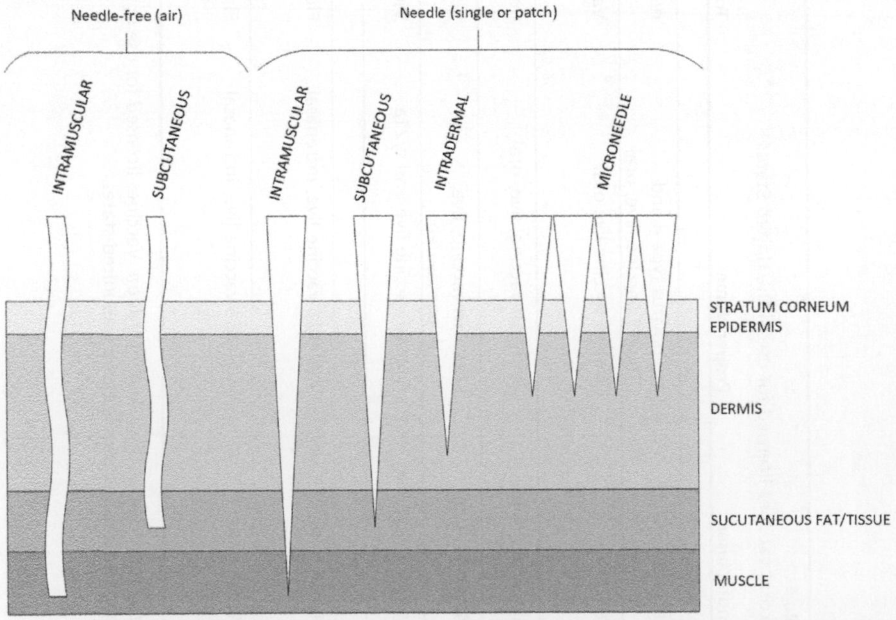

Fig. 1. Visual representation of vaccine delivery depth by method of delivery. (Created using Visio by the author.)

electrical current. Microneedles deliver the medication or vaccination into the dermal layer with less pain than experienced in typical subcutaneous injections.[31]

There are four different types of microneedles[32]:

- Solid microneedles for skin pretreatment to increase skin permeability
- Microneedles coated with drug that dissolves off in the skin
- Polymer microneedles that encapsulate drug and fully dissolve in the skin
- Hollow microneedles for drug infusion into the skin

Microneedles are typically used as a patch with the size and density of needles on the patch varying depending on the dose needed, but they can also be used in a single-needle delivery device.

Microneedles have been used to deliver whole, inactivated virus; trivalent split antigen vaccines; and DNA plasmids encoding the influenza hemagglutinin to rodents, and strong antibody responses were elicited. Several vaccines have been studied using microneedle delivery systems.

No serious adverse events or infections have been observed in trials using microneedle delivery systems. Although bleeding was a concern, for short needles (<1 mm) there is little to no bleeding observed. Although other common injection side effects, such as redness and pain, have been observed, the pain has been reported as less than hypodermic needle injections.[32]

Needleless Delivery Systems/Air Gun

Needleless delivery systems for vaccine delivery have been used for mass vaccination campaigns since the 1940s.[33,34] Rather than using a hypodermic needle to penetrate the skin, a narrow stream under high pressure powered by compressed air or gas pushes the vaccine into the body. Immune responses following use of jet injectors have led to comparable or higher antibody titers compared with traditional injection.[26,35–37] Some limitations have included concerns about pain; site reactions, such as redness and swelling; and cross-contamination of other blood-borne infectious diseases, such as hepatis B and C and human immunodeficiency virus (HIV). Unlike older injector models that used a reusable head to deliver doses, newer versions use disposable heads and cartridge systems to reduce the risk of cross-contamination.[38]

EXPANDING USE OF VACCINES

Although acute infectious disease prevention remains the most common use of vaccination, newer technology combined with advanced understanding of disease mechanisms is opening the door for vaccines to prevent and manage a host of other diseases.

ONGOING CHALLENGES IN VACCINE DEVELOPMENT

Human Immunodeficiency Virus

Advances in HIV treatment and management have extended the lives of persons infected with HIV and preventive care using pre-exposure prophylaxis with effective antiretroviral therapy persons who are at high risk of HIV acquisition is considered standard of care by the US Preventive Services Task Force.[39,40] Researchers around the world have been working since 1987 to identify a vaccine capable of preventing HIV infections. Despite creating numerous candidates leveraging multiple mechanism and delivery systems, there is still no vaccine able to crease sustainable and protective protection against HIV.[40]

Hepatitis C

The burden of hepatitis C infection remains a global challenge and prevention through a multimodal approach is welcomed. Similar to HIV, hepatitis C infection treatment has advanced with improved morbidity and mortality because of direct-acting antiviral medication development, access, and use. Primary hepatitis C virus infection does not generate sterilizing immunity and research continues to struggle to develop an effective preventive vaccine.[41]

EMERGING DISEASES

Ebola Hemorrhagic Fever

Ebola disease or Ebola hemorrhagic fever is a viral hemorrhagic disease that on average kills 50% of those infected within 2 weeks. Passed through direct contact with infected bodily fluids, it spreads rapidly in outbreaks. More than 20 vaccine candidates have been developed with eight either in clinical trials or expected to begin clinical trials in the near future. In 2018 nearly 180,000 people in Congo received the recombinant vesicular stomatitis virus–Zaire Ebola virus (rVSV-ZEBOV) as a compassionate use of an experimental vaccine.[42] As the outbreak continues to spread across the Democratic Republic of the Congo a second vaccine candidate, Ad26.ZEBOV/MVA-BN Ebola Zaire, has been approved for use in a large-scale research trial beginning in August 2019.

Zika Virus

Zika virus is a mosquito-borne flavivirus that causes outbreaks of a congenital syndrome in fetuses of pregnant women characterized by microcephaly, craniofacial disproportion, spasticity, ocular abnormalities, and miscarriage. Infected adults typically experience an acute mild febrile illness, but some develop autoimmune dysfunction, such as Guillain-Barré syndrome.[43] Because Zika virus is related to other flaviviruses, such as Dengue virus, researchers have been able to use similar vaccine development strategies. Zika virus vaccine candidates are being developed as inactivated, subunit, and live-attenuated vaccines. There are currently around 20 vaccine candidates being pursued with some in clinical phase I/II trials. Three phase 1 clinical studies demonstrating safety and immunogenicity for inactivated and DNA subunit Zika virus vaccines were published.[44–46]

VACCINATING AGAINST NONINFECTIOUS DISEASES AND CONDITIONS

Expanding Use of the Bacillus Calmette-Guérin Vaccine

For more than 100 years an attenuated *Mycobacterium bovis* bacillus Calmette-Guérin (BCG) strain has been used as a vaccine against tuberculosis. In animal models BCG vaccine has shown promise against a range of inflammatory and autoimmune conditions including allergic asthma, multiple sclerosis, and type 1 diabetes.[47] A randomized 8-year-long prospective examination of subjects with type 1 diabetes with long-term disease who received two doses of the BCG vaccine showed lowered hemoglobin A_{1C} to near normal at Year 3 and the result persisted for the next 5 years.[48] BCG has also been used for many decades as a treatment of early stage noninvasive bladder cancer.[49]

Cancer Prevention and Treatment

Vaccines are used in cancer care for prevention and treatment of cancer. Two FDA-approved vaccines have been shown to effectively prevent cancer by preventing chronic infection with viruses associated with cancer development. Human papilloma virus vaccine has been shown to prevent cervical, vaginal, vulvar, and anal cancer, and is also suspected to reduce oral pharyngeal cancers.[50,51] Hepatis B vaccine has been shown to reduce hepatocellular carcinoma associated with chronic hepatitis B infection.[52]

Immunotherapy leverages the immune system's ability to attack and remove foreign antigens causing a particular disease. Although it is used for treating an existing infection, immunotherapy using therapeutic vaccination is an effective cancer treatment strategy. Autologous cancer vaccines are derived from the individual's immune or cancer cells. Although numerous autologous tumor cell vaccines have been studied, none has been successful enough to be FDA approved.[53] Dendritic cell vaccines have been more successful with more than 200 clinical trials demonstrating safety, immunogenicity, and ability to activate an antitumor response leading to clinically identifiable tumor regression.[54,55] There is one FDA-approved autologous dendritic cell vaccine used for treating prostate cancer. Sipuleucel-t (Provenge) has been shown in clinical trials to extend life for men with treatment-resistant metastatic prostate cancer.[56] Another dendritic cell vaccine against breast cancer is showing promise for women with HER-2-positive ductal carcinoma in situ.[55]

Allogenic cancer vaccines are created from nonself or laboratory-generated cancer cells. They offer a potentially cheaper and more accessible method for treated cancers with vaccination. Clinical trials are underway for vaccine treatments against bladder, brain, breast, colorectal, lung, renal, leukemia, melanoma, pancreatic cancers, and others. Many vaccine candidates are in development. None are currently available for clinical use.

SUMMARY

Vaccine science continues to evolve newer and safer ways to deliver prevention and treatment of infectious and noninfectious diseases. This includes new adjuvants to enhance immunogenicity; delivery systems to reduce pain and improve acceptability; and a wider range of uses including emerging infectious diseases, such as Zika virus and Ebola, and treatment of chronic diseases, such as cancer and autoimmune disorders.

DISCLOSURE

The author has nothing to disclose.

REFERENCES

1. Boylston A. The origins of inoculation. J R Soc Med 2012;105(7):309–13.
2. Pead PJ. Benjamin Jesty: new light in the dawn of vaccination. Lancet 2003;362:2104–9.
3. Edsall G. Smallpox vaccination vs inoculation. JAMA 1964;190(7):689–90.
4. Riedel S. Edward Jenner and the history of smallpox and vaccination. Proc (Bayl Univ Med Cent) 2005;18(1):21–5.
5. Hamilton JL. Vaccine science and immunology. In: Rockwell DOP, editor. Vaccine science and immunization guideline. Cham (Switzerland): Springer; 2017. p. 41–71.
6. Alving CR, Peachman KK, Rao M, et al. Adjuvants for human vaccines. Curr Opin Immunol 2012;24(3):310–5.

7. Centers for Disease Control and Prevention. Vaccine safety common concerns. Available at: https://www.cdc.gov/vaccinesafety/concerns/adjuvants.html. Accessed August 10, 2019.
8. Didierlaurent AM, Morel S, Lockman L, et al. AS04, an aluminum salt- and TLR4 agonist-based adjuvant system, induces a transient localized innate immune response leading to enhanced adaptive immunity. J Immunol 2009;183(10):6186–97.
9. Scheiermann J, Klinman DM. Clinical evaluation of CpG oligonucleotides as adjuvants for vaccines targeting infectious diseases and cancer. Vaccine 2014;32:6377.
10. Jackson S, Lentino J, Kopp J, et al. Immunogenicity of a two-dose investigational hepatitis B vaccine, HBsAg-1018, using a toll-like receptor 9 agonist adjuvant compared with a licensed hepatitis B vaccine in adults. Vaccine 2018;36(5):668–74.
11. Halperin SA, Ward B, Cooper C, et al. Comparison of safety and immunogenicity of two doses of investigational hepatitis B virus surface antigen co-administered with an immunostimulatory phosphorothioate oligodeoxyribonucleotide and three doses of a licensed hepatitis B vaccine in healthy adults 18-55 years of age. Vaccine 2012;30:2556.
12. Heyward WL, Kyle M, Blumenau J, et al. Immunogenicity and safety of an investigational hepatitis B vaccine with a Toll-like receptor 9 agonist adjuvant (HBsAg-1018) compared to a licensed hepatitis B vaccine in healthy adults 40–70 years of age. Vaccine 2013;31:5300.
13. Oxman MN, Levin MJ, Shingles Prevention Study Group. Vaccination against herpes zoster and postherpetic neuralgia. J Infect Dis 2008;197(Suppl 2):S228–36.
14. Gabutti G, Valente N, Sulcaj N, et al. Evaluation of efficacy and effectiveness of live attenuated zoster vaccine. J Prev Med Hyg 2014;55(4):130–6.
15. Levin MJ, Weinberg A. Immune responses to zoster vaccines. Hum Vaccin Immunother 2019;15(4):772–7.
16. Weinberg A, Kroehl ME, Johnson ME, et al. Comparative immune responses to licensed herpes zoster vaccines. J Infect Dis 2018;218(suppl_2):S81–7.
17. Dooling KL, Guo A, Patel M, et al. Recommendations of the Advisory Committee on Immunization Practices for Use of Herpes Zoster Vaccines. MMWR Morb Mortal Wkly Rep 2018;67:103–8.
18. Wallis J, Shenton DP, Carlisle RC. Novel approaches for the design, delivery and administration of vaccine technologies. Clin Exp Immunol 2019;196(2):189–204.
19. Prosper N. Boyaka. Inducing mucosal IgA: a challenge for vaccine adjuvants and delivery systems. J Immunol 2017;199(1):9–16.
20. Kim SH, Jang YS. The development of mucosal vaccines for both mucosal and systemic immune induction and the roles played by adjuvants. Clin Exp Vaccin Res 2017;6(1):15–21. https://www.ncbi.nlm.nih.gov/pmc/articles/PMC5292352/.
21. Federal Drug Administration. Vaccines licensed for use in the United States. Available at: https://www.fda.gov/vaccines-blood-biologics/vaccines/vaccines-licensed-use-united-states. Accessed August 10, 2019.
22. Riese P, Sakthivel P, Trittel S, et al. Intranasal formulations: promising strategy to deliver vaccines. Expert Opin Drug Deliv 2014;11(10):1619–34.
23. Jia Y, Krishnan L, Omri A. Nasal and pulmonary vaccine delivery using particulate carriers. Expert Opin Drug Deliv 2015;12(6):993–1008.
24. Ono A, Azukizawa H, Ito S, et al. Development of novel double-decker microneedle patches for transcutaneous vaccine delivery. Int J Pharm 2017;532(1):374–83.

25. Leone M, Mönkäre J, Bouwstra JA, et al. Dissolving microneedle patches for dermal vaccination. Pharm Res 2017;34(11):2223–40.
26. Shin CI, Jeong SD, Rejinold NS, et al. Microneedles for vaccine delivery: challenges and future perspectives. Ther Deliv 2017;8(6):447–60.
27. Herndon TO, Gonzalez S, Gowrishankar TR, et al. Transdermal microconduits by microscission for drug delivery and sample acquisition. BMC Med 2004;2:12.
28. Kalia YN, Naik A, Garrison J, et al. Iontophoretic drug delivery. Adv Drug Deliv Rev 2004;56:619–58.
29. Schoellhammer CM, Blankschtein D, Langer R. Skin permeabilization for transdermal drug delivery: recent advances and future prospects. Expert Opin Drug Deliv 2014;11:393–407.
30. Baxby D. Smallpox vaccination techniques; from knives and forks to needles and pins. Vaccine 2002;20(16):2140–9.
31. Gill HS, Denson DD, Burris BA, et al. Effect of microneedle design on pain in human volunteers. Clin J Pain 2008;24(7):585–94.
32. Prausnitz MR, Mikszta JA, Cormier M, et al. Microneedle-based vaccines. Curr Top Microbiol Immunol 2009;333:369–93.
33. Li N, Peng LH, Chen X, et al. Transcutaneous vaccines: novel advances in technology and delivery for overcoming the barriers. Vaccine 2011;29(37):6179–90.
34. Matsuo K, Hirobe S, Okada N, et al. Frontiers of transcutaneous vaccination systems: novel technologies and devices for vaccine delivery. Vaccine 2013;31(19):2403–15.
35. Fisch A, Cadilhac P, Vidor E, et al. Immunogenicity and safety of a new inactivated hepatitis A vaccine: a clinical trial with comparison of administration route. Vaccine 1996;14:1132–6.
36. Williams J, Fox-Leyva L, Christensen C, et al. Hepatitis A vaccine administration: comparison between jet-injector and needle injection. Vaccine 2000;18:1939–43.
37. Parent du Chatelet I, Lang J, Schlumberger M, et al. Clinical immunogenicity and tolerance studies of liquid vaccines delivered by jet-injector and a new single-use cartridge (Imule): comparison with standard syringe injection. Imule Investigators Group. Vaccine 1997;15:449–58.
38. Giudice EL, Campbell JD. Needle-free vaccine delivery. Adv Drug Deliv Rev 2006;58(1):68–89. https://doi.org/10.1016/j.addr.2005.12.003.
39. Final Recommendation Statement: Prevention of human immunodeficiency virus (HIV) infection: preexposure prophylaxis. U.S. Preventive Services Task Force. 2019. Available at: https://www.uspreventiveservicestaskforce.org/Page/Document/RecommendationStatementFinal/prevention-of-human-immunodeficiency-virus-hiv-infection-pre-exposure-prophylaxis. Accessed June 16, 2020.
40. Girard MP, Osmanov S, Assossou OM, et al. Human immunodeficiency virus (HIV) immunopathogenesis and vaccine development: a review. Vaccine 2011;29(37):6191–218. https://doi.org/10.1016/j.vaccine.2011.06.085.
41. Bailey J, Barnes E, Cox AL. Approaches, progress, and challenges to hepatitis C vaccine development. Gastroenterology 2019;156(2):418–30. https://doi.org/10.1053/j.gastro.2018.08.060.
42. World Health Organization. E. bola vaccine. Available at: https://www.who.int/ebola/drc-2018/faq-vaccine/en/. Accessed August 10, 2019.
43. Shan C, Xie X, Shi PY. Zika virus vaccine: progress and challenges. Cell Host Microbe 2018;24(1):12–7.
44. odjarrad K, Lin L, George SL, et al. Preliminary aggregate safety and immunogenicity results from three trials of a purified inactivated Zika virus vaccine

candidate: phase 1, randomised, double-blind, placebo-controlled clinical trials. Lancet 2018;391(10120):563–71.
45. Pantoja P, Perez-Guzman EX, Rodriguez IV, et al. Zika virus pathogenesis in rhesus macaques is unaffected by pre-existing immunity to dengue virus. Nat Commun 2017;8:15674.
46. Pardi N, Hogan MJ, Pelc RS, et al. Zika virus protection by a single low-dose nucleoside-modified mRNA vaccination. Nature 2017;543(7644):248–51.
47. Kowalewicz-Kulbat M, Locht C. BCG and protection against inflammatory and auto-immune diseases. Expert Rev Vaccin 2017;16(7):1–10.
48. Available at: https://www.nature.com/articles/s41541-018-0062-8. Accessed June 16, 2020.
49. Fuge O, Vasdev N, Allchorne P, et al. Immunotherapy for bladder cancer. Res Rep Urol 2015;7:65–79.
50. Gillison ML, Chaturvedi AK, Lowy DR. HPV prophylactic vaccines and the potential prevention of noncervical cancers in both men and women. Cancer 2008; 113(10 Suppl):3036–46.
51. Saslow D, Castle PE, Cox JT, et al. American Cancer Society Guideline for human papillomavirus (HPV) vaccine use to prevent cervical cancer and its precursors. CA Cancer J Clin. 2007;57:7–28.
52. Lim SG1, Mohammed R, Yuen MF, et al. Prevention of hepatocellular carcinoma in hepatitis B virus infection. J Gastroenterol Hepatol 2009;24(8):1352–7.
53. Goldman B, DeFrancesco L. The cancer vaccine roller coaster. Nat Biotechnol 2009;27(2):129–40.
54. Santos P, Butterfield LH. Dendritic cell–based cancer vaccines. J Immunol 2018; 200(2):443–9.
55. Palucka K, Banchereau J. Dendritic-cell-based therapeutic cancer vaccines. Immunity 2013;39(1):38–48.
56. Handy CE, Antonarakis ES. Sipuleucel-T for the treatment of prostate cancer: novel insights and future directions. Future Oncol 2018;14(10):907–17.

Impact of Human Papillomavirus Vaccination in Reducing Cancer

Mina S. Khan, MD[a], Margot Savoy, MD, MPH, FABC, CPE, CMQ[b,*]

KEYWORDS

• Vaccine • Immunization • HPV • HPV vaccine • Human papilloma virus
• Cervical cancer • Anogenital cancer

KEY POINTS

- Human papilloma virus is a significant cause of global morbidity and mortality, including cancers of the cervix, anus, oropharynx, and penis, leading many to focus on using vaccination as a key strategy for eradication.
- HPV vaccination is routinely recommended at age 11 and 12 years old and can be caught up through age 45 years.
- Giving a strong recommendation and conveying the safety of the vaccine are 2 effective strategies for encouraging HPV vaccination.

INTRODUCTION

Only 13 years have passed since the introduction of the first vaccine to prevent human papillomavirus the United States. Over the years, the composition and timing have evolved, but we are already beginning to see the expected results, including a significant drop in cervical intraepithelial neoplasia grades 2 or 3.[1] Although the news is promising, recent analysis by the Centers for Disease Control and Prevention (CDC) of the 2018 National Immunization Survey-Teen (NIS-Teen) show we still have work to do.[2] Coverage with at least 1 dose of HPV vaccine increased from 65.5% to 68.1%, and the percentage of teens up-to-date with a complete HPV vaccine series increased from 48.6% to 51.1%; however, these improvements were seen only in male individuals.[2] These data are similar to the results seen in the Healthy People 2020 (HP2020) tracking, whereas of 2017, the percentage of girls age 13 to 15 who have completed the 2-vaccine HPV series has risen to 49.9, and in boys this has

[a] Family Medicine, Primary Care Services-Blount, LLC, 101 Lemley Drive, Suite A, Oneonta, AL 35121, USA; [b] Family & Community Medicine, Temple Faculty Practice, Lewis Katz School of Medicine at Temple University, 1316 West Ontario Street, Room 310, Philadelphia, PA 19140, USA
* Corresponding author.
E-mail address: Margot.Savoy@tuhs.temple.edu

Prim Care Clin Office Pract 47 (2020) 529–537
https://doi.org/10.1016/j.pop.2020.05.007
0095-4543/20/

increased to 42.3. At the current rate of increase in vaccine uptake, the HP2020 80% goal will not likely be achieved, the increase in vaccine coverage is certainly a positive indicator.[3]

THE BURDEN OF HUMAN PAPILLOMAVIRUS

HPV is a double-stranded DNA virus with more than 100 genotypes, found only in humans. Of these genotypes, 13 are considered to be carcinogenic (HPV 16, 18, 31, 33, 35, 39, 45, 51, 52, 56, 58, and 59), and one has been classified as probably carcinogenic (HPV 68).[4] Genotypes HPV 16 and HPV 18 are responsible for approximately 70% of cervical cancer and cervical dysplasia worldwide. Low-risk genotypes, including HPV 6 and HPV 11, have been associated with the development of anogenital warts.[5] HPV is transmitted mainly through direct skin-to-skin or skin-to-mucosa contact and is the most common sexually transmitted infection in the United States.

Anogenital and Oropharyngeal Cancers

After breast, colorectal, and lung cancers, cervical cancer is the fourth most prevalent cancer in women. In the United States alone, it was predicted that 12,990 women would be diagnosed with cervical cancer in 2016, and 4120 would die from the disease.[6] According to the World Health Organization, newly diagnosed cases of cervical cancer in less developed countries contribute to 84% of the total global burden of cervical cancer. Similarly, approximately 311,000 women died of cervical cancer in 2018, with more than 85% of these occurring in low-income and middle-income countries.[7] The burden of HPV-related cancers goes beyond the cervix, with approximately 90% of anal cancers; 50% of vulvar, vaginal, and penile cancers; and 20% to 30% of oropharyngeal cancers being attributed to HPV infection.[8] In the United States, there were an estimated 8300 new cases of anal cancer; 2700 among men, and 5530 among women.[9]

Genital Warts

Anogenital warts are the most common clinical manifestation of HPV infection. The lesions are benign, although various distressing physical manifestations, including pain, bleeding, and itching may occur. Genital warts also can be a predictor for concurrent infection with high-risk oncogenic HPV genotypes. Low-risk genotypes, including HPV 6 and 11 are responsible for 97% of genital wart manifestations. In the United States, 5.6% of sexually active men and women ages 18 to 45 years have self-reported a diagnosis of genital warts; the incidence is estimated to be highest among men younger than 30 and decreases with age.[10]

SCREENING AND DIAGNOSIS OF HUMAN PAPILLOMAVIRUS INFECTION AND ITS SEQUELAE

Cervical Cytology and Human Papillomavirus Testing

Cervical cancer screening dates back to the 1940s, with the introduction of the Papanicolaou smear (Pap smear). Conventional cytology involves obtaining a specimen from the cervix and fixing directly on to a slide; this has been mostly replaced by liquid cytology in which the sampling device is stirred into a vial of preservative. The latter has been found to produce less unsatisfactory specimens, although some studies suggest no increase in sensitivity with this technique. In the late 1970s and early 1980s, HPV was identified as the causative agent in virtually all cases of cervical cancer worldwide. Most HPV infections and the low-grade lesions associated with them are transient and resolve spontaneously. The addition of molecular HPV testing for high-risk HPV types to the Pap smear helps determine whether any low-grade lesions warrant further diagnostic evaluation via colposcopy.[11]

In populations where participation in physician-directed or midwife-directed Pap smears is low, self-sampling of vaginal fluid for high-risk HPV types may be an option. There are limitations to this technique; despite the test's high sensitivity, the specificity is poor, and a high number of women identified with high-risk HPV will actually have no cytologic abnormalities on further testing. However, keeping in mind that the prevalence of high-risk HPV infections decreases with age, the specificity may approach that of Pap smear testing when performed in postmenopausal women.[12]

The US Preventive Services Task Force (USPSTF) revised its screening guidelines in 2018. The rationale behind the revision of the guidelines was the decline in number of deaths from cervical cancer since the introduction of widespread cervical cancer screening. Between 1975 and 2010, the incidence of cervical cancer has decreased by more than 50%.[13] Screening for cervical cancer should be performed every 3 years with cervical cytology alone in women aged 21 to 29 years. For women aged 30 to 65 years, screening is recommended every 3 years with cervical cytology alone, every 5 years with high-risk human papillomavirus (hrHPV) testing alone, or every 5 years with hrHPV testing in combination with cytology (Grade A recommendation).[11] The USPSTF discourages testing in women younger than 21 and older than 65, as well as in women who have undergone a hysterectomy with removal of the cervix, and do not have a prior history of a high-grade precancerous lesion or cervical cancer (Grade D recommendation).[14] These recommendations have been endorsed by the American Cancer Society, American Society for Colposcopy and Cervical Pathology, and American Society for Clinical Pathology, as well as by the American College of Obstetricians and Gynecologists.[15]

Anal Cytology and High Resolution Anoscopy

Because of similarities between cervical and anal cancer, similar screening techniques can be applied to both conditions. Screening for anal cancers can be performed via anal Pap smear, a technique that was introduced in the 1990s. Sensitivity and specificity have been shown to be similar to the cervical Pap smear, and HPV testing can also be performed when liquid-based cytology is obtained via digital rectal examination. Another screening modality is high resolution anoscopy, where a colposcopic examination of the anus is performed after application of 3% acetic acid, similar to cervical colposcopy. Lesions can be identified based on clinical impressions, and biopsies may be obtained.

Unlike screening for cervical cancer, there is no consensus on routine screening for anal cancer in the general population, either nationally or internationally. The disease is much less prevalent, hence routine screening is not cost-effective. In addition, no randomized clinical trials have been completed that might suggest improved morbidity and mortality among routinely screened individuals. However, there are certain populations at higher risk for developing anal cancer, and epidemiologic data suggest that screening for high-grade anal dysplasia in these populations may be cost-effective for early detection. Individuals at higher risk of developing anal dysplasia and cancer include adults infected with human immunodeficiency virus, particularly men who have sex with men, those with a history of condylomata, solid organ transplant recipients, and women with cervical or vulvar dysplasia. The New York State Department of Health AIDS Institute is one regional organization that recommends routine annual examination of the anus in these high-risk populations.[9,13]

Oral Screening

HPV causes an estimated 30,000 cases of oropharyngeal cancers worldwide and is becoming the major cause of these cancers in developed countries, with tobacco-related cases of head and neck squamous cell cancers on the decline. Because of the rising prevalence, there have been efforts to create a reliable screening method to detect early oropharyngeal cancers. One of the techniques used in detection of oral HPV involves oral rinsing. In a study conducted at Sloan Kettering University Cancer Center in New York, patients with a confirmed diagnosis of an oropharyngeal cancer were compared with a control group with no prior diagnosis, using a qualitative test for detection of high-risk HPV in oral rinse specimens. The study concluded that the test was highly specific (98%) and potentially sensitive (79%) for oropharyngeal cancers and may have potential as a useful screening tool for early detection.[16]

THE HUMAN PAPILLOMAVIRUS VACCINE IN EVOLUTION

In June 2006, a quadrivalent vaccine called Gardasil, manufactured by Merck and Co., was licensed by the Food and Drug Administration (FDA) for use in the United States, for prevention of cervical cancer and genital warts in female individuals age 9 to 26. The vaccine was offered as a 3-dose schedule (0, 1–2, and 6 months). The genotypes targeted were 16 and 18, which are responsible for most cases of cervical cancer, and 6 and 11, which contribute to more than 90% of cases of anogenital warts. Licensure was followed by recommendations by the Advisory Committee on Immunization Practices (ACIP) to incorporate Gardasil into the vaccine schedule.[17] Subsequently, in October 2009, the bivalent vaccine, Cervarix, manufactured by GlaxoSmithKline was approved by the ACIP for use in female individuals age 9 to 25 for prevention of cervical cancer.[18] It was also concluded that Gardasil may be used in male individuals age 9 to 26 for prevention of genital warts, but ACIP did not recommend routine immunization at that time.

In December 2010, the FDA approved Gardasil for prevention of anal cancer, and this was followed in October 2011 by the ACIP's recommendation to routinely use the vaccine in male individuals age 9 to 21. The target age to initiate the series was 11 to 12 with catch-up vaccinations from age 13 to 21.[19]

After the approval of the 9-valent vaccine Gardasil-9 in 2015, the use of quadrivalent Gardasil declined, as did the demand for Cervarix. In October 2016, the ACIP immunization schedule was updated to reflect the use of the 9-valent vaccine.[20] Cervarix was eventually removed from the market because of low demand and is no longer available in the United States. Similarly, the distribution of quadrivalent Gardasil ceased in 2017.

In October 2018, the FDA approved the expanded use of Gardasil-9 to individuals age 27 to 45 not previously vaccinated. Supporting data were reviewed during subsequent ACIP meetings, and in June 2019, the age of catch-up immunizations was extended to all individuals up to age 26.[21] The committee also recommended shared clinical decision making regarding catch-up immunization for women and men age 27 to 45, but no changes have been made to the routine vaccination schedule to date.[21]

GLOBAL IMPACT OF HUMAN PAPILLOMAVIRUS VACCINATION STRATEGIES

HPV vaccine is currently licensed in more than 100 countries, including Europe, Australia, Canada, the United States, and increasingly in lower-income and middle-income countries. Currently more than 100 countries and territories include HPV vaccine in their immunization programs, and nearly 40 additional low-income and middle-income countries will begin soon. Although all countries have included a focus on immunization of teen girls ideally before sexual debut, the approach toward older women, boys, and men has varied. Used of school-based strategies appear to be quite effective across high-income, middle-income, and low-income countries. Studies have found that school-based models have been effective in demonstration programs in Malaysia, Peru, Uganda, Vietnam, and India (vaccine coverage ranged from 82.6% to 96.1%).[22,23] These highly effective programs are important because in countries with vaccination coverage of at least 50%, a 65% decline in HPV 16/18 was observed.[24]

Australia

Australia was an early adopter of HPV vaccination. The National HPV Vaccination Program launched in 2007 and initially included both a funded school-based program for girls at age 12 to 13 years and a community-based program for women up to age 26. Australia transitioned to a gender-neutral program in 2013 by extending the funded program to include boys aged 12 to 13 years and catch-up for boys aged 14 to 15 years through 2014. In January 2018 the program transitioned to using the 2-dose course of the nonavalent vaccine. The national program is already showing signs of success. The Vaccine Impact in Population study was completed in a sentinel site comparing women 18 to 24 years who presented to the clinic for Pap testing. The prevalence of infection with 4vHPV vaccine types declined from 28.7% in 2005 to 2007 to 2.3% (2010–2012) ($P<.0001$).[25] In addition to lower prevalence rates, declining rates of high-grade cervical abnormalities, genital warts, and incidence of juvenile-onset recurrent respiratory papillomatosis have been observed.[26]

Rwanda

Before 2011 neither HPV vaccination nor cervical cancer screening were easily accessible in private or governmental clinics in Rwanda. A school-based vaccination program with no out-of-pocket costs was implemented and resulted in 92% to 95% coverage for girls in primary grade 6.[27] Although the program was not without its challenges, key factors in Rwanda's successful implementation included government ownership and support for the program, school-based delivery, social mobilization, and strategies for reaching out-of-school girls.

BARRIERS TO HUMAN PAPILLOMAVIRUS IMMUNIZATION

A number of barriers to HPV vaccination have been identified including cost/financing the vaccine, inadequate supply and vaccine access, lack of knowledge about vaccine safety and effectiveness, and resistance to vaccination.[28] Across studies, parents consistently list a strong recommendation by their health care professional as one of the most important factors in their decision to vaccinate. Aside from general factors that reduce vaccine uptake in certain populations, there are also hurdles specific to the HPV vaccine.

Parental Factors

In the United States, women living below the poverty line are 3 times more likely to be infected with high-risk HPV, and also experience higher morbidity and mortality secondary to sequelae of the virus. There are higher rates of cervical cancer in Hispanic and African American women, which may be a consequence of lower rates of Pap testing and poorer adherence to follow-up guidelines following an abnormal Pap smear. Unfortunately, this group is more likely to have lower family income, which is a strong predictor of access to health care.[29]

Race/Ethnicity

Various studies have addressed barriers to HPV vaccine coverage among historically underserved populations; these have found that African American and Hispanic girls are less likely to receive a recommendation for the vaccine from a health care professional, and also are less likely to complete the series compared with non-Hispanic white girls.[28] Parents may have limited knowledge about HPV and availability of the vaccine because of not receiving a robust recommendation from a health care professional.

Cultural beliefs

Parents who are aware of the availability of the HPV vaccine may still not understand how their children could benefit. They might believe that their children are too young to be vaccinated, because they are not yet sexually active, or have concerns that vaccinating their child against HPV could be interpreted as condoning sexual activity. They may also be reluctant to discuss the vaccine's purpose with their child, which could necessitate discussion about sexual activity.[29] This is often considered a taboo subject, particularly in younger adolescents.

The impact of media

The HPV vaccine has received both negative and positive coverage in conventional and social media. A study of information derived from Twitter revealed a strong correlation between misrepresentation of the HPV vaccine on the platform, and vaccine acceptance rates, independent of socioeconomic factors, suggesting that consumption of social media may impact a parent's decision whether or not to vaccinate their child.[28] In another study, parents who had heard only negative stories about the HPV vaccine either on social media, or in conventional media, were less likely to have initiated or completed the HPV vaccine series for their children. Interestingly, in the same study it was observed that parents who had only been exposed to positive coverage about the HPV vaccine expressed more intention to have their children vaccinated, but this did not necessarily translate into higher uptake of the vaccine.[30,31]

Health Care Professionals

Knowledge gaps

Some studies have discussed a lack of knowledge among health care professionals regarding the association between HPV and genital warts or cancers of sites other than the cervix, which may lead to clinicians choosing a perceived risk-based approach, only, for example, not offering the vaccine to male individuals because they may not be aware of the benefits. Concerns among health care professionals about safety have been rarely identified as a barrier to offering the HPV vaccine.[29]

Cost and reimbursement

For physicians not participating in their state's Vaccines for Children program, stocking the vaccine may be cost prohibitive, particularly if reimbursement by insurance companies is delayed.

Parental attitudes

Health care professionals cite parents' attitudes toward the HPV vaccine as a barrier, which is often compounded by time constraint when trying to address additional health needs of the adolescent.

Table 1
Selected resources to facilitate human papillomavirus vaccination conversations

Title	Organization	Web Site
HPV for Clinicians	Centers for Disease Control and Prevention	https://www.cdc.gov/hpv/hcp/index.html
How I Recommend Videos	Centers for Disease Control and Prevention	https://www.cdc.gov/vaccines/howirecommend/index.html
Vaccine Conversations with Parents	Centers for Disease Control and Prevention	https://www.cdc.gov/vaccines/hcp/conversations/index.html
National HPV Vaccination Roundtable	Coalition of >70 organizations	https://hpvroundtable.org/
National AHEC Organization HPV Project	National AHEC (Area Health Education Center)	https://www.nationalahec.org/index.php/what-we-do/national-training-center/hpv-project/resources-for-health-professionals
Human Papilloma Virus	American Cancer Society	https://www.cancer.org/cancer/cancer-causes/infectious-agents/hpv.html
Vaccines for Teens	American Academy of Family Physicians	https://www.aafp.org/patient-care/public-health/immunizations/vaccines-teens.html

Several online resources have been developed by various organizations to help facilitate the discussion regarding the HPV vaccine between parents and physicians. These include audiovisual aids, and printable materials, and some can be found in **Table 1**.

THE FUTURE OF HUMAN PAPILLOMAVIRUS VACCINATION

The ability to vaccinate against HPV is already having an impact on the incidence of infection and HPV-associated cancers. As major organizations and countries look to eradicate HPV-related cancers, scientists continue to work to develop new and even more effective vaccines.[32] Targeted HPV-related cancer therapy using vaccines is being studies and may provide a promising approach to reducing morbidity and mortality.[33] In the meantime, using effective strategies to encourage early immunization at 11 to 12 years old is our best hope for eradicating HPV-related diseases and cancers in the world.

DISCLOSURE

The authors have nothing to disclose.

REFERENCES

1. McClung NM, Gargano JW, Bennett NM, et al. Trends in human papillomavirus vaccine types 16 and 18 in cervical precancers, 2008–2014. Cancer Epidemiol Biomarkers Prev 2019. https://doi.org/10.1158/1055-9965.EPI-18-0885.

2. Walker TY, Elam-Evans LD, Yankey D, et al. National, regional, state, and selected local area vaccination coverage among adolescents aged 13-17 years-United States, 2018. MMWR Morb Mortal Wkly Rep 2019;68:718–23.
3. Healthy People 2020. Infectious diseases. 2019. Available at: https://www.healthypeople.gov/2020/topics-objectives/topic/immunization-and-infectious-diseases/objectives. Accessed September 25, 2019.
4. International Agency for Research on Cancer. Human papillomaviruses, 2018. Lyon (France): International Agency for Research on Cancer; 2018.
5. Steben M, Garland S. Genital warts. Best Pract Res Clin Obstet Gynaecol 2014;28:1063–73.
6. Yoo W, Kim S, Huh W, et al. Recent trends in racial and regional disparities in cervical cancer incidence and mortality in United States. PLoS One 2017;12(2):E0172548.
7. Human papillomavirus (HPV) and cervical cancer. World Health Organization; 2019. Available at: https://www.who.int/en/news-room/fact-sheets/detail/human-papillomavirus-(hpv)-and-cervical-cancer. Accessed August 10, 2019.
8. Moscicki A. Impact of HPV infection in adolescent populations. J Adolesc Health 2005;37:S3–9.
9. Berry M, Jay N. High resolution anoscopy. In: Pfenninger J, Fowler C, editors. Pfenninger and Fowler's procedures for primary care. 3rd edition. Philadelphia: Elsevier Mosby; 2011. p. 677–84.
10. Anic G, Giulano A. Genital HPV infection and related lesions in men. Prev Med 2011;53:S36–41.
11. Safaeian M, Solomon D, Castle P. Cervical cancer prevention—cervical screening: science in evolution. Obstet Gynecol Clin North Am 2007;34(4):739–60.
12. Wikstrom J, Lindell M, Sanner K, et al. Self-sampling and HPV testing or ordinary pap-smear in women not regularly attending screening: a randomized study. Br J Cancer 2011;105:337–9.
13. Leeds I, Fang S. Anal cancer and intraepithelial neoplasia screening: a review. World J Gastrointest Surg 2016;8(1):41–51.
14. Grade Definitions. US Preventive Services Task Force website. 2018. Available at: https://www.uspreventiveservicestaskforce.org/Page/Name/grade-definitions. Accessed August 10, 2019.
15. US Preventive Services Task Force. Screening for cervical cancer, US Preventive Services Task Force recommendation statement. JAMA 2018;320(7):674–86.
16. Centers for Disease Control and Prevention. Cervical cancer screening guidelines for average-risk women. 2019. Available at: https://www.cdc.gov/cancer/cervical/pdf/guidelines.pdf. Accessed August 15, 2019.
17. Rosenthal M, Huang B, Katabi N, et al. Detection of HPV related oropharyngeal cancer in oral rinse specimens. Oncotarget 2017;8(65):109393–401.
18. Centers for Disease Control and Prevention. FDA licensure of bivalent human papillomavirus vaccine (HPV2, Cervarix) for use in females and updated HPV vaccination recommendations from the Advisory Committee on Immunization Practices (ACIP). Morb Mortal Wkly Rep 2010;59(20):626–9.
19. Centers for Disease Control and Prevention. FDA licensure of quadrivalent human papillomavirus vaccine (HPV4, gardasil) for use in males and guidance from the Advisory Committee on Immunization Practices (ACIP). Morb Mortal Wkly Rep 2010;59(20):630–2.

20. Petrosky E, Bocchini J, Hariri S, et al. Use of 9-valent human papillomavirus (HPV) vaccine: updated HPV vaccination recommendations of the Advisory Committee on Immunization Practices. Morb Mortal Wkly Rep 2015;64(11):300–4.
21. Meites E, Szilagyi PG, Chesson HW, et al. Human papillomavirus vaccination for adults: updated recommendations of the Advisory Committee on Immunization Practices. Morb Mortal Wkly Rep 2019;68:698–702.
22. Muhamad NA, Buang SA, Jaafar S, et al. Achieving high uptake of human papillomavirus vaccination in Malaysia through school-based vaccination programme. BMC Public Health 2018;18(1):1402.
23. Friedman AL, Oruko KO, Habel MA, et al. Preparing for human papillomavirus vaccine introduction in Kenya: implications from focus-group and interview discussions with caregivers and opinion leaders in Western Kenya. BMC Public Health 2014;14:855.
24. Drolet M, Bénard É, Boily MC, et al. Population-level impact and herd effects following human papillomavirus vaccination programmes: a systematic review and meta-analysis. Lancet Infect Dis 2015;15(5):565–80.
25. Tabrizi SN, Brotherton JM, Kaldor JM, et al. Assessment of herd immunity and cross-protection after a human papillomavirus vaccination programme in Australia: a repeat cross-sectional study. Lancet Infect Dis 2014;14(10):958–66.
26. Patel C, Brotherton JM, Pillsbury A, et al. The impact of 10 years of human papillomavirus (HPV) vaccination in Australia: what additional disease burden will a nonavalent vaccine prevent? Euro Surveill 2018;23(41):1700737.
27. Binagwaho A, Wagner C, Gatera M, et al. Achieving high coverage in Rwanda's national human papillomavirus vaccination programme. Bull World Health Organ 2012;90:623–8.
28. Holman DM, Benard V, Roland KB, et al. Barriers to human papillomavirus vaccination among US adolescents: a systematic review of the literature. JAMA Pediatr 2014;168(1):76–82.
29. Downs L, Scarini I, Einstein M, et al. Overcoming the barriers to HPV vaccination in high-risk populations in the US. Gynecol Oncol 2010;117:486–90.
30. Margolis M, Brewer N, Shah P, et al. Stories about HPV vaccine in social media, traditional media and conversations. Prev Med 2019;118:251–6.
31. Dunn A, Surian D, Leask J, et al. Mapping information exposure on social media to explain differences in HPV vaccine coverage in the United States. Vaccine 2017;35:3033–40.
32. Kumar S, Biswas M, Jose T. HPV vaccine: current status and future directions. Med J Armed Forces India 2015;71(2):171–7.
33. Kawana K, Adachi K, Kojima S, et al. Therapeutic human papillomavirus (HPV) vaccines: a novel approach. Open Virol J 2012;6:264–9.

Vaccine Policy in the United States

John W. Epling, MD, MSEd

KEYWORDS

- Vaccine • Immunization • Health policy • Vaccine hesitancy • Public health
- Guideline

KEY POINTS

- Vaccine safety and efficacy are ensured by the US Food and Drug Administration, the Centers for Disease Control and Prevention, the National Vaccine Program, and a robust safety monitoring program.
- Vaccine recommendations are made by the Advisory Committee on Immunization Practices, an advisory committee to the director of the Centers for Disease Control and Prevention, and recommendations are harmonized for use by all clinical specialties in the United States.
- The National Vaccine Program and National Vaccine Advisory Committee ensure coordination between the companies and public agencies involved in vaccine production.
- Vaccine laws attempt to balance the ethical principles in public health law and are the focus of much change and scrutiny.

INTRODUCTION

Vaccination is consistently touted as one of the top 10 most influential public health achievements in the United States.[1,2] Rates of vaccine-preventable communicable diseases have plummeted since the introduction of vaccines in the early to mid twentieth century. This degree of success has led the vaccine manufacturers and public health agencies into the realms of cancer and chronic illness prevention (eg, with the human papillomavirus [HPV] and hepatitis B vaccines) as a result of the decreased communicable disease burden. However, these gains are increasingly threatened. Expressions of reasonable concern about vaccine safety and effectiveness have now developed into growing communities of distrust in science and public health. Vaccines work best with a combination of strong immunogenicity in individuals and widespread adoption of vaccines by communities. Because vaccine protection is never 100% effective, society relies on this "herd immunity" to prevent the spread of disease in our communities. Recently, the increase in the number of recommended vaccinations,

Department of Family and Community Medicine, Virginia Tech Carilion School of Medicine, 1 Riverside Circle, Suite 102, Roanoke, VA 24016, USA
E-mail address: jwepling@carilionclinic.org

Prim Care Clin Office Pract 47 (2020) 539–553
https://doi.org/10.1016/j.pop.2020.05.011
primarycare.theclinics.com

the fading collective memory of the diseases we have successfully suppressed, and the availability of social networks that recklessly reinforce confirmation biases has caused segments of the population to reevaluate the risk–benefit calculation of vaccines.

Primary care clinicians practice on the front lines of these changes. Low vaccine rates in practice have roots in a lack of provider understanding of vaccine recommendations, safety monitoring, and public health law and economic issues.[3–5] A better understanding of the development of vaccines, vaccine recommendations and the interaction of federal agencies, federal and state laws, and specialty societies concerning vaccines can enable the practicing primary care clinician to conduct knowledgeable conversations with their patients about vaccine recommendations and safety concerns.

This article reviews the process of vaccine licensure, vaccine guideline development, vaccine funding, and vaccine-related public health law. The focus of this overview is on organizations and policies that influence primary care delivery of vaccines.

ADVISORY COMMITTEE ON IMMUNIZATION PRACTICES

Organization and Structure

The most relevant vaccine policy organization for primary care clinicians is the Advisory Committee on Immunization Practices (ACIP) of the Centers for Disease Control and Prevention (CDC). The role of the ACIP is to advise the director of the CDC and the secretary of the Department of Health and Human Services about the clinical use of vaccinations in the United States and to determine coverage recommendations for the Vaccines for Children Program (VFC). The ACIP is composed of 15 voting members who serve 4-year terms, chosen by the secretary of the Department of Health and Human Services on the recommendation of the ACIP steering committee. The membership includes one lay member. The committee must include at least 20% minority (black or African American, Hispanic, American Indian/Alaska native, or Asian) membership. Potential members are either nominated by professional organizations or self-nominated. In-depth expertise in vaccines and immunization is the principal requirement for membership.[6–8]

Organizing and providing support for the ACIP are the secretariat and the steering committee staffed by the CDC. The steering committee members provide support to the ACIP workgroups and meet before each ACIP meeting to discuss the agenda, membership, and other logistical matters.[6–8]

The ACIP is led by a chair, selected from the membership by the ACIP steering committee, who serves a 3-year term. There are several ex officio members of the ACIP who also vote on immunization recommendations, and a number of nonvoting liaison affiliate members, who represent stakeholder organizations such as medical professional societies and other interested parties. The ACIP is organized under the statute governing federal advisory committees; there is a robust conflict of interest policy, the meetings must be open to the public, and the reports and transcripts of the meetings are made public.[6–9]

The ACIP workgroups are created to perform a large amount of the preparatory and postrecommendation work for the ACIP. There must be 2 ACIP voting members on each workgroup, a CDC staff member, and (for vaccine-specific workgroups) a liaison from the US Food and Drug Administration (FDA). The remainder of the workgroup usually includes liaisons from various clinical societies and consultants as appropriate. Representatives from pharmaceutical manufacturers may attend workgroup meetings to provide necessary information about a topic, but may be asked to leave during any discussions of the topic. The workgroup meetings (usually held by teleconference) are closed working meetings of the ACIP, and, as such, formal deliberations on ACIP recommendations do not occur in workgroups. Vaccine-specific workgroups review data and help the CDC staff member to construct the presentations made to the ACIP in support of their deliberations. Other workgroups are involved in the logistics of organizing and presenting the schedules, and in evaluating best immunization practices and combination vaccines. The ACIP workgroups as of May 2019 are shown in **Box 1**.[6]

The process of an ACIP recommendation may involve several meetings at which a particular vaccine is reviewed and discussed. Once a vaccine is licensed by the US FDA for use (either a new license, or an expanded indication, age group, etc), the ACIP begins its work to evaluate its recommendation. Work on the vaccine begins in the vaccine-specific workgroups, led by ACIP members and CDC staff. The workgroups, on their regular teleconferences, hear the scientific data on the burden of disease, the safety and effectiveness of the vaccine, the FDA indications, and any applicable health economic data.[10] The workgroup deliberates the evidence and arrives at proposed recommendations and workgroup considerations for presentation and discussion at the in-person ACIP meetings. At this meeting, the workgroup chair and CDC staff present the introduction and background for the vaccine, the evidence review, applicable economic information, the evidence-to-recommendations framework (new as of 2010, discussed elsewhere in this article), and the workgroup commentary and proposed recommendations. Public comment, a required component of any federal advisory committee, is solicited, followed by a vote on the proposed recommendation. The vote can be for a routine or general recommendation (A), for a permissive or shared decision-making recommendation (B), or no recommendation. Once a recommendation is approved, it becomes official upon its publication in the CDCs *Morbidity and Mortality Weekly Report (MMWR)*.[11]

Box 1
ACIP workgroups (as of May 2019)

Adult Immunization Schedule

Child/Adolescent Immunization Schedule

General Best Practices

Influenza Vaccines

Combination Vaccines

Dengue Vaccine

Hepatitis Vaccines

Herpes Zoster Vaccines

Human papillomavirus (HPV) Vaccines

Meningococcal Vaccines

Pneumococcal Vaccines

RSV Vaccines—Pediatric

Pertussis Vaccines

Rabies Vaccines

From Centers for Disease Control and Prevention. ACIP work groups. Available at: https://www.cdc.gov/vaccines/acip/workgroups.html.

The ACIP's General Best Practices Committee workgroup discusses broader clinical, implementation and feasibility issues with vaccines—general contraindications and precautions, adverse reaction prevention and management, vaccine administration issues, record keeping, immunocompetency, and other emerging vaccination issues that do not clearly belong to an existing workgroup. This group maintains and revises the *General Best Practices Guidelines for Immunization*—known informally as the "Pink Book"—a useful reference to assist with the implementation of vaccine recommendations in practice.[12]

The ACIP's workgroups on the Adult and Child/Adolescent Immunization Schedules review the recent recommendations from the ACIP and incorporate them into the schedules that serve as the principal method for communicating vaccine recommendations to clinicians. The committees ready the schedules for publication on the CDC website, and in select clinical journals. The ACIP limits the number of publication partners for the schedules to decrease the possibility of error between publications of the schedules. The schedules contain graphical, color-coded tables showing age and condition-based timelines for vaccinations. In addition, the "Notes" section of the schedules contains important dosing and indication information for each vaccine in the schedule.

Example: Expanding the Recommendations for Human Papillomavirus 9 Vaccine

The processes of the ACIP is best understood through an example. In early October 2018, the FDA expanded the indications for 9-valent HPV vaccine to men and women aged 27 through 45 years old. This expansion was based on a study of 3200 women aged 27 to 45 years that showed a decrease in a composite end point that included genital warts; vulvar, vaginal, and cervical precancerous lesions; and persistent HPV infection, as well as HPV-related invasive cervical cancer. In addition, the FDA considered observational evidence from long-term follow-up of earlier vaccinated cohorts. The effectiveness for men was based on an inference from the data from women, a small 150-subject study in men aged 27 to 45 years examining immunogenicity data, and extrapolation of efficacy data from the men 16 to 26 years of age. The FDA also examined safety in 13,000 men and women, revealing relatively minor adverse effects.[13]

In late October 2018, the expanded HPV indications were first discussed in an ACIP meeting, along with some reassuring safety data concerning a lack of association of HPV vaccine with primary ovarian insufficiency. Recommendation options were reviewed at that meeting, but the workgroup continued to review the evidence—bringing the topic back to the February 2019 meeting for additional review and discussion. At this meeting, more detailed health economic and statistical modeling data were reviewed, as well as the results of program and vaccine provider surveys. Finally, in June 2019 the summary of the available evidence and health economic models was reviewed, as well as the evidence-to-recommendations framework. The evidence-to-recommendations framework, published on the ACIP website, notes the elements of the ACIP's decision making and concerns with this expanded recommendation.[14] The ACIP noted some uncertainty about the acceptability of HPV vaccine in this cohort owing to some conflicting evidence, although the general acceptance of HPV vaccination was felt to be high. They wrestled with the issue of expanding a recommendation in the setting of a current global shortage of vaccine owing to inadequate production capacity. In the discussion concerning the feasibility of the recommendation, there was conflicting concern about whether a general recommendation in this age group could ameliorate or worsen vaccination disparity, depending on the availability of insurance. After considering this framework, public comments were heard, and the final vote was held, resulting in a B recommendation (a recommendation based on shared decision making between the patient and the provider) for both men and women in the 27- through 45-year-old age group. This recommendation, as per ACIP procedure, became official upon its publication in the MMWR in August 2019.[11,15]

Evolution of the Advisory Committee on Immunization Practices

Before 1995, the ACIP produced its own vaccine schedule, as did the American Academy of Pediatrics (AAP) and the American Academy of Family Physicians (AAFP). In 1995, there arose differences in recommendations between the AAP and the ACIP concerning the timing of the second MMR vaccine dose. This potential for confusion around differing recommendations led to collaboration between the ACIP and the clinical specialty organizations—AAFP, AAP, and the American College of Physicians to produce a "harmonized" vaccine schedule. The schedule is produced by the ACIP, with input from specialty organizations through the workgroups and ACIP liaisons, and then the schedule is adopted by the specialty organizations. This system has worked well since 1995, with only minor exceptions—such as preferences for certain forms of vaccine over others—occurring recently.

The ACIP's process for making vaccine recommendations has always included a review of the burden of disease, an understanding of the vaccine's effectiveness, and a rigorous assessment of its safety and health economic data. In 2010, the ACIP implemented an explicit process to transparently document the process of reaching their recommendations. It selected the GRADE framework,[16] which has been adopted by a large number of international guideline-producing organizations and includes the development and review of an evidence-to-recommendations framework as an agenda item with each vaccine topic requiring a vote. This framework examines the quality of the body of evidence that informs a given clinical recommendation—rating its strength based on risk of bias (including publication bias), precision, applicability, consistency, strength of association, evidence of a dose–response relationship, and impact of potential bias. The ACIP recognizes that there is not always the opportunity to conduct a well-designed randomized controlled trial to understand the effectiveness of vaccines—especially when the public health threat is rapidly emerging—but this framework makes the decision-making process systematic and explicit. Less ideal study designs may be used by the ACIP to understand the postrecommendation impact of the vaccine, examine long-term outcomes, and so on. The GRADE framework also allows the incorporation of information and judgment derived from an examination of patient values and from health economic data.[10] The ACIP did not adopt the final "strong/weak" recommendation description of the GRADE approach, but kept its A, B, and no recommendation categories.[17,18]

The February 2019 release of the ACIP's Adult and Child/Adolescent Immunization Schedules debuted extensive formatting and wording changes. As a result of 2 years of usability testing, end-user interviews, and work with consulting human factors engineers, the adult and child schedules were changed to improve readability and consistency and to decrease word count. The goal of the changes was to communicate clear recommendations and provide concise clinical data in the notes sections to support clinicians' vaccination practice.[19]

NATIONAL VACCINE PROGRAM AND NATIONAL VACCINE ADVISORY COMMITTEE

The National Vaccine Program (NVP) is a less commonly known agency in the government whose functions are to promote vaccine development and research; ensure the appropriate licensing of vaccinations for safety and efficacy; ensure adequate production, supply, and distribution of vaccines across the country; and monitor adverse effects related to vaccinations. The NVP is part of the Office of Infectious Disease and HIV/AIDS, in the Office of the Assistant Secretary of Health in the Department of Health and Human Services. The NVP coordinates and provides direction to the multiple federal agencies involved in vaccine development, licensing, recommendation, supply, and distribution, including the National Institutes of Health, the CDC, the FDA office of Biologics Research and Review, the Department of Defense, and the Agency for International Development.

The NVP supports and convenes the National Vaccine Advisory Committee, which is composed of members "from among individuals who are engaged in vaccine research or the manufacture of vaccines or who are physicians, members of parent organizations concerned with immunizations, or representatives of State or local health agencies or public health organizations." The National Vaccine Advisory Committee commissions research and advises the director of the NVP on the functions as listed, recommending and prioritizing the efforts of the NVP.

The NVP created, in 2010, the US National Vaccine Plan.[20] This plan had 5 overarching goals:

1. Develop new and improved vaccines
2. Enhance the vaccine safety system
3. Support communications to enhance informed vaccine decision-making
4. Ensure a stable supply of, access to, and better use of recommended vaccines in the United States
5. Increase global prevention of death and disease through safe and effective vaccination

In 2016, the NVP conducted a planned midcourse review of the National Vaccine Plan.[21] This review noted good progress across all the Plan's objectives, listing multiple achievements in each of the 5 focus areas. The review also recommended the following "opportunity areas" for further focus:

- Strengthen health information and surveillance systems to track, analyze, and visualize disease, immunization coverage, and safety data, both domestically and globally.
- Foster and facilitate efforts to strengthen confidence in vaccines and the immunization system to increase coverage rates across the lifespan.
- Eliminate financial and systems barriers for providers and consumers to facilitate access to routine, recommended vaccines.
- Strengthen the science base for the development and licensure of vaccines.
- Facilitate vaccine development.

The Office of Infectious Disease and HIV/AIDS manages an umbrella website, vaccines.gov, which is a useful compilation of links and information about vaccines, including clinical information, vaccine availability and resources, and vaccine safety.

THE FOOD AND DRUG ADMINISTRATION CENTER FOR BIOLOGICS EVALUATION AND RESEARCH

Before a vaccine can be recommended for clinical use, it must be approved and licensed for use by the FDA. The Center for Biologics Evaluation and Research is the FDA center responsible for recommending such approval based on a phased research system that is very similar to that required for pharmaceuticals. The vaccine manufacturer (sponsor) submits an Investigational New Drug application to the FDA with preliminary safety and immunogenicity information as well as the results of any animal testing and presents its plan for human trials. Phase I studies examine safety and immunogenicity in small groups of human subjects (usually tens of subjects). Phase II studies examine the efficacy of different doses, usually requiring hundreds of subjects. The phase III studies are the largest, involving thousands of subjects, and usually report both immunogenicity and clinical outcome effectiveness data as well as important safety outcomes. If there are any concerns about the vaccine's safety or efficacy during this process, the FDA reserves the right to request additional study to answer those questions. Once sufficient study data are obtained, the sponsor requests licensure. The FDA review team considers the available data and inspects the proposed manufacturing facilities before approval. In addition, the sponsor and the FDA may choose to have their data reviewed by the Vaccines and Related Biological Products Advisory Committee—a group of non-FDA clinical and research experts, and including a consumer representative—who will additionally advise the FDA on the safety and effectiveness of the vaccine for the submitted indication.[22]

Once a vaccine is approved, the FDA has responsibility for continued oversight of production of at the sponsor's facilities, through regulations and inspections. An important ongoing vaccine safety measure includes the phase IV studies of vaccine safety required after licensure for most vaccines. The FDA has ex officio liaison representation to the ACIP and close communication, through the NVP, to other federal agencies responsible for vaccine development and recommendation.[22]

VACCINES FOR CHILDREN AND IMMUNIZATION QUALITY IMPROVEMENT FOR PROVIDERS

Given the public health importance of the vaccination of children against common communicable diseases, the US government has created a system to ensure that children who are uninsured or underinsured can be fully vaccinated. The VFC was created by congress in the Omnibus Reconciliation Act of 1993 as a reaction to the measles epidemics in the early 1990s. The CDC had determined that more than one-half of the children who contracted measles in these outbreaks had not been vaccinated, despite many of them having seen a health care provider. VFC provides free vaccines to children (through age 18) who are Medicaid eligible, uninsured, underinsured, or American Indian/Alaskan Native. Children whose insurance covers vaccines, even if the insurance includes a deductible, are not eligible. In some cases, children must be seen at Federally Qualified Health Centers or Rural Health Clinics to receive VFC vaccines, but for most children, their own health care providers can enroll in the VFC program. There are significant regulations concerning the receipt, storage, and administration of federally funded VFC vaccine in practices. Accurate logging, specific vaccine storage requirements, and strict inventory control are required for participation in the program. The VFC program is generally regarded as a significant success, increasing vaccine rates across the country and reducing racial and ethnic disparities in vaccination rates, and, on average, decreasing income-based disparities.[23,24]

IMMUNIZATION INFORMATION SYSTEMS

Immunization information systems (IIS) are the most available example of an attempt to integrate the infrastructures of clinical care and public health. Accurate record keeping of vaccines administered to a patient has benefits for both the patient and society. IIS, previously known as immunization registries, are regional or state-wide electronic databases of vaccinations administered to patients. Data can be uploaded by any vaccination provider and can be downloaded by an approved vaccine information user—schools, public health departments, and other clinical providers. These systems have evolved from regional systems that required written informed consent by each patient recorded in the system to now state-wide registries with either a mandate for participation or implied consent with an opt-out policy for both adults and children. IIS are covered entities under the Health Insurance Privacy and Portability Act owing to their role in public health.[25–28]

The use of an IIS is required for participation as a VFC provider, and there are various other incentives and technologies being built around the use of these systems—the Meaningful Use incentives developed as part of the American Reinvestment and Recovery Act in 2009, clinical decision support programs, and vaccine barcoding systems. The CDC, who coordinates and administers the various IIS-associated programs, has clear strategic priorities involving IIS to enhance the delivery of vaccines in practice, improve the flow of vaccine-related clinical information to providers, coordinate the technology standards needed to improve the systems, and improve the ability of the IIS to help target public health activities to increase immunization rates. Research on the implementation of these systems has found benefits for audit and feedback strategies to increase provider vaccine delivery rates and cost savings owing to increased administrative efficiency.[27,29–31] However, there remain gaps in use by primary care physicians owing to problems with communication between the IIS and the electronic health record, and difficulty with updating the IIS electronically.[32] A national IIS does not seem to be on the immediate horizon, but the improved integration of IIS within the electronic health records along with the development of accurate clinical decision support promise to further expand on the established usefulness of these systems.

CLINICAL SPECIALTY SOCIETIES AND VACCINE POLICY

Despite the existence of national policies and guidance concerning immunizations, most primary care organizations have also weighed in on immunization policy. For clinical recommendations, any differences in policy have been minor, given the agreement on harmonization of the vaccine recommendations since 1995. However, each clinical society has a set of vaccine-related policies that focus on improving vaccination rates and supporting the information needs of providers and patients about vaccines.

The AAP is strongly focused on promoting vaccination and generally refers to the CDC/ACIP policies and recommendations.[33,34] This information is supported with additional information from the AAP's Red Book[35]—a well-regarded reference about the management of pediatric infectious diseases in practice. The AAP has convened, since 2008, the Immunization Alliance—a group of specialty societies and advocacy groups—to improve communication about the clinical and public health benefits of vaccines, to dispel inaccurate information about vaccines, and to advocate at all levels for science-based vaccine policy.[36]

The AAFP has specific policies that encourage the broad, low-cost availability of vaccines to the entire population. It advocates for first-dollar coverage for all immunizations and full funding of government vaccine programs to provide low- or no-cost vaccines to practices. To improve the family physician's ability to provide vaccines, the AAFP advocates for timely and equitable distribution of vaccine to family physicians, improving the flow of information about vaccine administration to the patient-centered medical home, and adequate economic support for vaccine provision in practices, including overhead costs associated with maintaining a vaccine inventory, and support for administration of the vaccines in practice. The AAFP sponsors a vaccine science fellowship, funded by an unrestricted educational grant from Merck, Inc., to develop a cadre of family physicians that are knowledgeable about vaccine science and policy to represent the AAFP on guideline and policy committees nationally. Finally, the AAFP has conducted Immunization Champion projects during which representatives from practices around the country collaborate on quality improvement initiatives to improve the rate of vaccine delivery in their practices.

The American College of Physicians has a similar quality improvement program for immunizations called "I Raise the Rates." This program provides resources for tracking vaccine rates in practice and reporting on the success of quality improvement initiatives through the American Board of Internal Medicine's Maintenance of Certification program. The American College of Physicians also has numerous policies supporting the use of immunizations, advocating for full vaccination of health care providers and advocating against nonmedical exemptions for vaccines.

With the increased recognition of the clinical importance of maternal vaccination during pregnancy, the American College of Obstetricians and Gynecologists has been very active in vaccination policy. It has convened a Maternal Immunization Task Force (with other maternity care provider organizations) to educate providers and advocate for greater rates of recommended maternal vaccination. It has also created a variety of programs and resources—recognition awards, educational products, resource toolkits, and so on—to support and promote their campaign "Immunization for Women."

Among nonprimary care societies, the Infectious Disease Society of America[4,37] and the National Foundation for Infectious Diseases[38] are both leaders in vaccine policy and promotion. The Immunization Action Coalition[4,39] and the National Adult and Influenza Immunization Summit[40] are 2 of the leading nongovernmental, non–specialty-related organizations promoting vaccines and vaccination policy and help government agencies and specialty societies to coordinate their vaccine advocacy efforts.

VACCINATION LAW AND EXEMPTION POLICIES

Few topics in health care have aroused the level of controversy in recent years like vaccine law and vaccination exemption.[41] Requiring vaccination in certain key settings has been a cornerstone of successful public health policy for decades. Recently, however, the phenomenon of vaccination hesitancy has challenged this success. The most effective examples of mandatory vaccination are the requirements for schools and day cares, colleges, and health care facilities. Schools and day cares tend to have the broadest requirements, requiring essentially full compliance with age-based ACIP vaccination recommendations upon entry. As children age, the requirements tend toward more focus on acutely communicable public health threats for those age groups, for example, TdaP vaccine for 11-year-olds to boost pertussis immunity, MCV4 vaccine to reduce meningococcal incidence in settings where crowding can occur including college dormitories, military barracks, and others. HPV vaccination, in addition to the other challenges to its acceptance, is often perceived as an extension of the concept of protection against communicable disease, because of the measure of behavioral choice that moderates the risk of exposure to HPV. As a result, some states have exempted HPV from mandatory vaccine requirements. For health care workers, mandatory vaccination is meant not only for personal protection of the health care workers, but to increase herd immunity to protect patients seeking care in the facility. Typically mandated or encouraged vaccinations for health care workers are those most frequently associated with health care facility outbreaks, namely, TdaP, hepatitis B, MMR, and influenza. A recent epidemic of hepatitis A infection in Appalachia spreading eastward has caused hospitals to offer and encourage hepatitis A vaccination for its most susceptible workers (environmental, food service, and emergency department staff).[42]

For public school and day care vaccination requirements, the states have been the locus of regulation. All states and the District of Columbia currently require vaccination for school and day care attendees.[43] In 4 states—Indiana, Michigan, Ohio, and South Dakota—it is unclear as to whether the same requirements apply to private schools.[44] Colleges generally set their own requirements based on best practice and on consultation with local and state public health officials. Health care facilities have generally set their own requirements, but states are beginning to regulate these requirements.[45] Even some national public health requirements are being added. For example, the CDC and the Centers for Medicare and Medicaid Services have collaborated on the National Healthcare Safety Network, a network of health care facilities working on decreasing the rate of health care-acquired infections. As a part of this effort, a seasonal influenza vaccine compliance rate of greater than 90% has been instituted as a financially incentivized performance measure for acute care hospitals.[46]

Exemptions from these site-based or legal requirements for vaccination fall into 3 generally accepted categories: medical, religious, and personal. Medical exemptions include any listed contraindication to the vaccine based on allergy, prior severe reaction, or immune status. Religious exemptions fall into 3 major categories: prohibition against taking a life, dietary laws, and interference with the natural order.[47] Personal or philosophic exemptions are more difficult to classify beyond simply documented preference or a history of a "strong personal conviction."

Over the past few decades, nonmedical exemption laws have increased.[48,49] Research has documented that the choice not to vaccinate not only puts the unvaccinated individual at risk, but also increases the likelihood of outbreaks of vaccine-preventable disease in that area and outbreak incidence has increased proportionally to the increase in nonmedical exemptions.[50–53]

Recognizing this risk, states are gradually tightening the regulations for exemptions. Many states have specific policies to exclude unvaccinated children from school during an outbreak situation, to revoke the exemption during an outbreak, or to require additional documentation before approving an exemption.[44] A few states are removing both personal and religious exemptions because of their experiences with outbreaks, most recently in areas of New York, where outbreaks in the generally unvaccinated Orthodox Jewish community have sickened hundreds.[54] Several reviews of the major religious teachings cited by those seeking vaccine exemptions conclude that, with the exception of Christian Science, all major religions accommodate and encourage the use of vaccination to preserve health.[47,55] Recent reviews of legal approaches to promoting parental compliance with school vaccination requirements finds no support for the right to vaccine exemption in the federal or state constitutions. These reviews list a number of legal approaches that balance the ethical principles of autonomy, beneficence, and justice that inform much of public health law. The approaches include persuasion through education, financial incentives or penalties, and various forms of legal and regulatory coercion.[56–63] There has even been a recent call for national vaccine exemption policy to constrain the variation between states because of the convenience and ease of travel between states.[64]

DISCUSSION

There is a broad and robust system for the support of clinical and public health vaccination strategies, including systems for licensure, safety monitoring, clinical recommendations, and data tracking. A coherent set of vaccination laws and policies is lacking, but because of the vaccine-preventable disease outbreaks in recent years, there is growing push for improvement. The estimated economic burden of vaccine preventable disease in this the United States, with our current vaccine rates, is still approximately $9 billion—80% of which is attributed to vaccine hesitancy.[64] It is the domain of state and national guidelines, policies, and laws to reduce the disease and expenditure associated with vaccine preventable disease.

The voice of primary care is increasingly needed in this area. Primary care clinicians can provide important knowledge, perspective, and advocacy for sound vaccination policy to improve our current system. As the ACIP evaluates newer vaccines for chronic diseases and cancer and for the less common infectious diseases, it will become increasingly important for primary care clinicians to have a working understanding of the ACIP methods so that they may optimally use what promise to be more nuanced and complex vaccine recommendations.[65] An appreciation of FDA regulations, vaccine financing, and data systems will enable the primary care clinician to take an active role in vaccine delivery and to advocate for any needed changes in our system.

DISCLOSURE

The author has nothing to disclose.

REFERENCES

1. Centers for Disease Control and Prevention. Ten Great Public Health Achievements – United States, 1900-1999. Available at: https://www.cdc.gov/mmwr/preview/mmwrhtml/00056796.htm. Accessed September 29, 2019.
2. Domestic Public Health Achievements Team, Centers for Disease Control and Prevention. Ten Great Public Health Achievements — United States, 2001–2010. Available at: https://www.cdc.gov/mmwr/preview/mmwrhtml/mm6019a5.htm. Accessed September 29, 2019.
3. Salmon DA, Pan WKY, Omer SB, et al. Vaccine knowledge and practices of primary care providers of exempt vs. vaccinated children. Hum Vaccin 2008;4(4):286–91.
4. Nichol KL, Zimmerman R. Generalist and subspecialist physicians' knowledge, attitudes, and practices regarding influenza and pneumococcal vaccinations for elderly and other high-risk patients: a nationwide survey. Arch Intern Med 2001;161(22):2702–8.
5. Hurley LP, Allison MA, Pilishvili T, et al. Primary care physicians' struggle with current adult pneumococcal vaccine recommendations. J Am Board Fam Med 2018;31(1):94–104.
6. Centers for Disease Control and Prevention. ACIP General Information | CDC. 2019. Available at: https://www.cdc.gov/vaccines/acip/committee/index.html. Accessed September 22, 2019.
7. Centers for Disease Control and Prevention. Advisory Committee on Immunization Practices (ACIP) Charter | CDC. 2019. Available at: https://www.cdc.gov/vaccines/acip/committee/charter.html. Accessed September 22, 2019.
8. Smith JC. Immunization policy development in the united states: the role of the advisory committee on immunization practices. Ann Intern Med 2009;150(1):45.
9. The Federal Advisory Committee Act. Available at: https://www.gsa.gov/policy-regulations/policy/federal-advisory-committee-management/legislation-and-regulations/the-federal-advisory-committee-act. Accessed September 22, 2019.

10. Centers for Disease Control and Prevention. ACIP Guidance for Health Economics Studies | CDC. 2019. Available at: https://www.cdc.gov/vaccines/acip/committee/economic-studies.html. Accessed September 28, 2019.
11. Centers for Disease Control and Prevention. ACIP Meeting Agenda Archive | CDC. 2019. Available at: https://www.cdc.gov/vaccines/acip/meetings/agenda-archive.html. Accessed September 28, 2019.
12. Ezeanolue E, Harriman K, Hunter P, et al. ACIP General Best Practice Guidelines for Immunization | Recommendations | CDC. 2019. Available at: https://www.cdc.gov/vaccines/hcp/acip-recs/general-recs/index.html. Accessed September 28, 2019.
13. Office of the Commissioner, Food and Drug Administration. FDA approves expanded use of Gardasil 9 to include individuals 27 through 45 years old. FDA. 2019. Available at: http://www.fda.gov/news-events/press-announcements/fda-approves-expanded-use-gardasil-9-include-individuals-27-through-45-years-old. Accessed September 28, 2019.
14. Centers for Disease Control and Prevention. EtR for HPV Vaccination of Adults 27-45 Years Old | CDC. 2019. Available at: https://www.cdc.gov/vaccines/acip/recs/grade/HPV-adults-etr.html. Accessed September 28, 2019.
15. Meites E. Human papillomavirus vaccination for adults: updated recommendations of the advisory committee on immunization practices. MMWR Morb Mortal Wkly Rep 2019;68. https://doi.org/10.15585/mmwr.mm6832a3.
16. Grade Working Group. GRADE home. Available at: http://gradeworkinggroup.org/. Accessed September 28, 2019.
17. Ahmed F, Temte JL, Campos-Outcalt D, et al, ACIP Evidence Based Recommendations Work Group (EBRWG). Methods for developing evidence-based recommendations by the Advisory Committee on Immunization Practices (ACIP) of the U.S. Centers for Disease Control and Prevention (CDC). Vaccine 2011;29(49):9171–6.
18. Lee G. Updated framework for development of evidence-based recommendations by the advisory committee on immunization practices. MMWR Morb Mortal Wkly Rep 2018;67. https://doi.org/10.15585/mmwr.mm6745a4.
19. Kim DK, Hunter P, on behalf of the Advisory Committee on Immunization Practices. Recommended Adult Immunization Schedule, United States, 2019. Ann Intern Med 2019;170(3):182.
20. Office of Infectious Disease and HIV/AIDS Policy (OIDP). U.S. National Vaccine Plan. HHS.gov. 2009. Available at: https://www.hhs.gov/vaccines/national-vaccine-plan/index.html. Accessed September 28, 2019.
21. Office of Infectious Disease and HIV/AIDS Policy (OIDP). 2010 National vaccine plan mid course review 2010. p. 58. Available at: https://www.hhs.gov/vaccines/national-vaccine-plan/midcourse/index.html. Washington, DC.
22. Center for Biologics Evaluation and Research. Vaccine product approval process. Silver Spring, MD: FDA; 2019. Available at: http://www.fda.gov/vaccines-blood-biologics/development-approval-process-cber/vaccine-product-approval-process. Accessed July 9, 2019.
23. Walsh B, Doherty E, O'Neill C. Since the start of the Vaccines for Children Program, uptake has increased, and most disparities have decreased. Health Aff (Millwood) 2016;35(2):356–64.
24. Centers for Disease Control and Prevention. VFC | About the Program | Vaccines for Children Program | CDC. 2019. Available at: https://www.cdc.gov/vaccines/programs/vfc/about/index.html. Accessed September 28, 2019.

25. Pabst LJ, Williams W. Immunization information systems. J Public Health Manag Pract 2015;21(3):225.
26. Williams W. Immunization Information Systems (IIS) Fundamentals: Overview and Development [Internet]. National Vaccine Advisory Committee Meeting; 2017 Jun 6 [cited 2020 Jun 21]; Washington, DC. Available at: https://www.hhs.gov/sites/default/files/Williams_IIS%20Fundamentals%20remediated.pdf.
27. Groom H, Hopkins DP, Pabst LJ, et al. Immunization information systems to increase vaccination rates: a community guide systematic review. J Public Health Manag Pract 2015;21(3):227.
28. Martin DW, Lowery NE, Brand B, et al. Immunization information systems: a decade of progress in law and policy. J Public Health Manag Pract 2015;21(3): 296–303.
29. Patel M, Pabst L, Chattopadhyay S, et al. Economic review of immunization information systems to increase vaccination rates: a community guide systematic review. J Public Health Manag Pract 2015;21(3):253.
30. Centers for Disease Control and Prevention. IIS | Home | Immunization Information Systems | CDC. 2019. Available at: https://www.cdc.gov/vaccines/programs/iis/index.html. Accessed September 28, 2019.
31. Murthy N, Rodgers L, Pabst L, et al. Progress in childhood vaccination data in immunization information systems — United States, 2013–2016. MMWR Morb Mortal Wkly Rep 2017;66(43):1178–81.
32. Kempe A, Hurley LP, Cardemil CV, et al. Use of immunization information systems in primary care. Am J Prev Med 2017;52(2):173–82.
33. American Academy of Pediatrics. Immunization strategies and practices: pediatric collection | AAP gateway. Available at: https://www.aappublications.org/iz sp. Accessed September 30, 2019.
34. American Academy of Pediatrics. Child vaccination across America. Available at: AAP.org http://www.aap.org/en-us/advocacy-and-policy/aap-health-initiatives/immunizations/Pages/Across-America.aspx. Accessed September 8, 2019.
35. AAP Committee on Infectious Diseases. Red book. Itasca, IL: American Academy of Pediatrics; 2018. Available at: https://ebooks.aappublications.org/content/9781610021470/9781610021470.
36. American Academy of Pediatrics. Immunization Alliance. AAP.org. Available at: http://www.aap.org/en-us/advocacy-and-policy/aap-health-initiatives/immunizations/Pages/Immunization-Alliance.aspx. Accessed September 30, 2019.
37. Infectious Disease Society of America. Immunization and vaccine policy. Available at: https://www.idsociety.org/policy–advocacy/immunization-and-vaccine-policy/. Accessed September 8, 2019.
38. National Foundation for Infectious Diseases. Vaccine science & safety—National Foundation for Infectious Diseases. Available at: https://www.nfid.org/immunization/vaccine-science-safety/. Accessed September 30, 2019.
39. Immunization Action Coalition. Immunization Action Coalition (IAC): vaccine information for health care professionals. Available at: https://www.immunize.org/. Accessed September 30, 2019.
40. National Adult and Influenza Immunization Summit |. Available at: https://www.izsummitpartners.org/. Accessed September 30, 2019.
41. Hendrix KS, Sturm LA, Zimet GD, et al. Ethics and childhood vaccination policy in the United States. Am J Public Health 2016;106(2):273–8.
42. Centers for Disease Control and Prevention. Outbreak-specific considerations for hepatitis A vaccine administration | CDC. 2019. Available at: https://www.cdc.

gov/hepatitis/outbreaks/InterimOutbreakGuidance-HAV-VaccineAdmin.htm. Accessed September 29, 2019.
43. State mandates on immunization and vaccine-preventable diseases. Available at: https://www.immunize.org/laws/. Accessed September 8, 2019.
44. Office for State, Tribal, Local and Territorial Support, Centers for Disease Control and Prevention. State School Immunization Requirements and Vaccine Exemption Laws [Internet]. Centers for Disease Control and Prevention; 2015 [cited 2020 Jun 21]. Available at: https://www.cdc.gov/phlp/docs/school-vaccinations.pdf.
45. Centers for Disease Control and Prevention. CDC - Vaccination Laws - Publications by Topic - Public Health Law. 2019. Available at: https://www.cdc.gov/phlp/publications/topic/vaccinationlaws.html. Accessed September 8, 2019.
46. Centers for Disease Control and Prevention. CMS - ACH Requirements | NHSN | CDC. 2019. Available at: https://www.cdc.gov/nhsn/cms/ach.html. Accessed September 29, 2019.
47. Grabenstein JD. What the World's religions teach, applied to vaccines and immune globulins. Vaccine 2013;31(16):2011–23.
48. Centers for Disease Control and Prevention. SchoolVaxView | Exemptions from State Vaccination Requirements | CDC. 2019. Available at: https://www.cdc.gov/vaccines/imz-managers/coverage/schoolvaxview/requirements/exemption.html. Accessed September 29, 2019.
49. National Conference of State Legislators. States with religious and philosophical exemptions from school immunization requirements. Available at: http://www.ncsl.org/research/health/school-immunization-exemption-state-laws.aspx#Table1. Accessed September 28, 2019.
50. Phadke VK, Bednarczyk RA, Salmon DA, et al. Association between vaccine refusal and vaccine-preventable diseases in the united states: a review of measles and pertussis. JAMA 2016;315(11):1149–58.
51. Bednarczyk RA, King AR, Lahijani A, et al. Current landscape of nonmedical vaccination exemptions in the United States: impact of policy changes. Expert Rev Vaccin 2019;18(2):175–90.
52. Wang E, Clymer J, Davis-Hayes C, et al. Nonmedical exemptions from school immunization requirements: a systematic review. Am J Public Health 2014;104(11):e62–84.
53. Olive J, Hotez P, Damania A, et al. The state of the antivaccine movement in the United States: a focused examination of nonmedical exemptions in states and counties. Available at: https://journals.plos.org/plosmedicine/article?id=10.1371/journal.pmed.1002578. Accessed September 28, 2019.
54. Pew Research Center. Amid measles outbreak, New York closes religious exemption for vaccinations – but most states retain it. Available at: https://www.pewresearch.org/fact-tank/2019/06/28/nearly-all-states-allow-religious-exemptions-for-vaccinations/. Accessed September 29, 2019.
55. Pew Research Center. Most in major U.S. religions support requiring childhood vaccination. Available at: https://www.pewresearch.org/fact-tank/2017/02/07/majorities-in-all-major-religious-groups-support-requiring-childhood-vaccination/. Accessed September 29, 2019.
56. Weithorn LA, Reiss DR. Legal approaches to promoting parental compliance with childhood immunization recommendations. Hum Vaccin Immunother 2018;14(7):1610–7.
57. Diekema DS. Personal belief exemptions from school vaccination requirements. Annu Rev Public Health 2014;35:275–92.

Printed and bound by CPI Group (UK) Ltd, Croydon, CR0 4YY
03/10/2024
01040465-0015

58. Salmon DA, Sapsin JW, Teret S, et al. Public health and the politics of school immunization requirements. Am J Public Health 2005;95(5):778–83.
59. Constable C, Blank NR, Caplan AL. Rising rates of vaccine exemptions: problems with current policy and more promising remedies. Vaccine 2014;32(16):1793–7.
60. Gostin LO, Ratzan SC, Bloom BR. Safe vaccinations for a healthy nation: increasing US vaccine coverage through law, science, and communication. JAMA 2019;321(20):1969–70.
61. Davis MM, Shah SK. Outbreaks of vaccine-preventable diseases: responding to system failure with national vaccination requirements. JAMA 2019;322(1):33–4.
62. Bylander J. The United States' piecemeal approach to vaccine policy. Health Aff (Millwood) 2016;35(2):195–8.
63. Office of the Commissioner, Food and Drug Administration. FDA Commissioner: Federal Government May Regulate Vaccines | Time. Available at: https://time.com/5534592/fda-commissioner-federal-government-vaccine-policies/. Accessed September 8, 2019.
64. Ozawa S, Portnoy A, Getaneh H, et al. Modeling the economic burden of adult vaccine-preventable diseases in the United States. Health Aff (Millwood) 2016;35(11):2124–32.
65. Bennett NM. The role of the Advisory Committee on Immunization Practices in ensuring optimal use of vaccines. JAMA 2019;321(4):341–2.